Purpose Driven Movement

A System for Functional Training

Acknowledgments

This book started with an idea. To make this idea a reality we sought out people within our circle of influence. Without their contributions, this undertaking would not have been possible.

Firstly, we want to thank our exceptional office support team and the world-class presenting team who have represented FTI with aplomb throughout the years.

Secondly, we want to extend a gracious shout out to:

- Steve Brossman, for helping us to take an idea and making it a reality.

- Ulrik Larson from Rehab Trainer, for writing much of Part 2 of this book, *Assess with Purpose,* and making it coherent and relevant to our theme.

- Dr Luke Delvecchio, for substantiating the theoretical portions of our 5 Pillars with the latest research.

- Jacq Ng, for providing a great perspective on personality typing and coaching.

- Our international partners: Mike Fitch of Animal Flow®; Tim Anderson of Original Strength; Dr Emily Splichel of Barefoot Trainer; Martin Rooney of Training for Warriors; Thomas Plummer; and Nick Winkelman.

Finally, our deep gratitude extends to those unsung who helped make this dream a reality.

First published in 2019 by Grammar Factory

© Tarek Michael-Chouja & Dan Henderson 2019
The moral rights of the author have been asserted

All rights reserved. Except as permitted under the *Australian Copyright Act 1968* (for example, a fair dealing for the purposes of study, research, criticism or review), no part of this book may be reproduced, stored in a retrieval system, communicated or transmitted in any form or by any means without prior written permission. All enquiries should be made to the author.

Printed in Australia by McPherson's Printing Group
Text design by Charlotte Gelin Design
Cover design by Designerbility
Editing by Grammar Factory

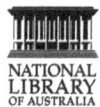 A catalogue record for this book is available from the National Library of Australia

Disclaimer

The material in this publication is of the nature of general comment only, and does not represent professional advice. It is not intended to provide specific guidance for particular circumstances and it should not be relied on as the basis for any decision to take action or not take action on any matter which it covers. Readers should obtain professional advice where appropriate, before making any such decision. To the maximum extent permitted by law, the author and publisher disclaim all responsibility and liability to any person, arising directly or indirectly from any person taking or not taking action based on the information in this publication.

To all those coaches over the years
who have instilled their coaching wisdom in a couple of Aussie blokes
seeking to better themselves –

We salute and thank you.

Tarek and Dan have really done something special with their book, *Purpose Driven Movement*. I believe that this book is an infinitely useful tool for both fitness professionals and fitness enthusiasts. What makes this book stand apart is the level of detail on everything from coaching practice to programming, while still being presented in a way that makes the techniques immediately applicable.

Mike Fitch, creator of *Animal Flow*®

This book ranks up there with the best of Dan John, Mike Boyle
and the other great coaches who have changed the way we think about training
through their philosophy and writings.

It was written by two true professionals, with decades of experience between them gained the hard way, one slogging mile after another on planes and working with fitness professionals in countries most of the rest of us only dream of visiting.

Dan Henderson and Tarek Michael-Chouja, founders of the
Functional Training Institute, have earned the right to create this book.
There can never be great writing in the fitness business unless the authors have paid their dues working with clients of all levels for a long number of years, and these two have dedicated most of their adult life to changing the world through fitness education, and this book reflects the best of what they have learned.

I started reading this new work late in the day and found myself still reading late into the night. It is well written, thoroughly researched and would be a must have addition to anyone's bookshelf who calls himself a fitness professional. Simply a great book by a couple of guys who have earned my respect in this business.

Thomas Plummer, author of *Soul of a Trainer*

A great training system will shift success from chance to choice. In Purpose Driven Movement, you will find just such a system. By design, this book lays out a blueprint that will simultaneously upgrade you as a designer of programs and a developer of people. All that's left is for you to read the book and your clients to reap the rewards.

Nick Winkelman, author of *Language of Coaching: the Art and Science of Movement*

Purpose Driven Movement provides one of the most comprehensive and integrative approaches to safe & effective programming. The intelligent flow of mobilisation and stabilisation sequences will empower all professionals to safely and effectively train a wide range of client demographics. This book is a must read for any and all health and fitness professionals.

Dr Emily Splichal, DPM, MS, founder of EBFA Global and author of *Barefoot Strong*

The careers of too many personal trainers and coaches are way too short. We need more trainers to pass that five-year mark when they really start to get good at training others. Following the program in this book will avoid many of the pitfalls common to people 'young' in the training business, and put them on a sustainable path to success.

Tom Myers, author of *Anatomy Trains*

Foreword

'A coach's purpose is
to help someone else find their own.'

One of the deepest questions a person can ask about his or her life is, 'What is my purpose?'

On the surface, that question may not sound so difficult to answer, but few people either invest the time to entertain it or have the courage to follow their findings once they have.

Why are you here?

What were you put on this earth to do?

Once you know the answer, you discover that your purpose acts as a compass and guides your every action.

Over the last two decades I have led my global fitness organization called Training for Warriors. In order to do that, I have used my own compass not only to direct the ship, but also to find and network with people on the same mission.

When you meet a person 'on purpose' you are immediately drawn to them. You listen to what they have to say. Because they are so clear about where they are going, you follow their lead.

Two people who clearly know their purpose are my friends Dan Henderson and Tarek Michael-Chouja.

When we first met over five years ago, I knew these Aussies were going to do something impactful in fitness. Their hunger to learn, network and grow was apparent. I had met a lot of people with those desires. But these two guys were different. Why? They weren't interested in growing for selfish reasons; they were interested in growing to grow other people.

After spending months in both the US and Australia with them, I know them as men serving a higher purpose in the fitness industry: they are dedicated to coach, educate and empower fitness professionals globally.

Unlike a number of companies trying to find the next silver bullet or weight loss trick, FTI was not created to fix just a few people for immediate benefit; it was created to help fix our industry. This book, which has taken them over three years to create, is their vehicle to serve that purpose.

Why would they take on such a huge endeavor as this book? Why would they painstakingly spend years researching and developing the content so you could improve? Simple. When you are living on purpose, you don't just want to do a thing, you're compelled to. And perhaps the most interesting part of being on purpose is that the things you do aren't tough; they are actually fun.

By reading this book, you will learn their training system (Adaptive Functional Training System) so you can enhance your understanding of what functional training is in the context of coaching, assessing, movement and programming. This is what they refer to as 'Purpose Driven Movement'.

I am sure you will agree the detail that has gone into this book makes it relevant, current and progressive. The research, collaboration, and contributors to the book only further enhance the credibility of the theme. Like other books, this book is informative, but the way it is interactive and supported by videos and photos to assist the reader in not only understanding functional training but also how to pursue it practically, make it unique.

I have heard the goal in life is to discover your gifts. If that is true, then one purpose of life is to give those gifts away.

Tarek and Dan have the gifts of curiosity, compassion and work ethic to make trainers and coaches better around the world. This book is a manifestation of their purpose, since they are giving those gifts to you.

Martin Rooney
Founder, Training for Warriors
Charlotte, North Carolina
2018

Contents

Introduction	17
The problem of dysfunctional 'functional training'	18
Introducing the Adaptive Functional Training System	23
Who is this book for?	30

Part 1: Coach with Purpose
– The Art and Science of Coaching

Coaching Foundations: The 3 Cs	33
Culture	36
Connection	45
Challenge	54
Coaching Technique: Cuing and Feedback	63
Cuing	64
Feedback	77
Conclusion	84

Part 2: Assess with Purpose
– Injury Awareness, Prevention and Monitoring

The Background Story on Fitness and Injuries	87
Injuries in fitness: what are the statistics?	89
How effective is injury prevention?	91
Injury screening and prediction	95
Are you injury aware?	97

Effective Injury Screening	99
The three layers of dysfunction	102
The injury prevention screen	111
Be a champion of injury prevention	119

Part 3: Move with Purpose – The 5 Pillars of Functional Training

Pillar 1 – Restore Function and Movement	123
Common questions	124
Warm-up activity	129
Joint rolling	129
Soft tissue work	130
Mobilisations and activations	131
Stretching	153
Mobility flows and movement prep	156
Pillar 2 – Develop Proper Movement Patterns	163
Bodyweight movement: sling systems and primal patterns	165
Suspended fitness	172
Crawling and Animal Flow®	176
Pillar 3 – Load the Foundations	187
Training the stabilisers of the body	187
The exercises	192
Pillar 4 – Build Strength and Power	209
Training with kettlebells	211
The exercises	216

Pillar 5 – Integrate Complex Movement Patterns	233
The battling rope	234
Progressions and complexes with the battling rope	238
Complexes with other tools	251

Part 4: Program with Purpose – Bringing it All Together

Programming Theory: Behind the Adaptive FTS	267
Understanding periodisation	268
The macrocycle/training plan	272
The mesocycle/training phase	275
The microcycle/sessions	276
Program review	285

The Adaptive FTS Program	287
Background information	287
Sample Adaptive FTS 12-Week Program	289
Adapting the program for different clients	299

Next steps	301

Resource pool	303
Coach with Purpose	303
Assess with Purpose	304
Move with Purpose	304
Program with Purpose	305

Introduction

Over the past ten years, functional training has moved from being a sideshow in the world of strength, conditioning and performance to an established and growing field of interest among fitness enthusiasts, personal trainers and scientific researchers.

Nowadays it is difficult to find trainers or coaches who don't claim to use and teach functional training. Yet this rising trend brings with it a confusing variety of opinions about what constitutes functional training.

Ask five fitness professionals what functional training is, and you will likely get five different responses.

Common definitions include:

- Exercises that are performed in multiple planes
- Exercises that are multi-joint
- Exercises that are performed on unstable surfaces
- Exercises that mimic everyday movements
- Exercises that directly replicate sporting movements and enhance sporting prowess

These definitions are quite different, and functional training cannot encapsulate all the above.

To define functional training clearly, we need to remember what 'function' means: something that is designed to have practical use. This means that the training needs to have a purpose. Now, practical use is itself a broad term, and the practical needs of a professional athlete will differ from a regular client who is usually aiming to get active, lose weight and look and feel good. As sport scientist and author of *Supertraining* Dr Mel Siff rightly points out, functional training is therefore context specific.[1] This is why one definition will not suit all.

The idea of practical use explains why one popular way to define functional training is as 'movement that makes daily activities easier to perform'. Most people want to train so they can move more freely and do things like squatting, pushing, pulling and twisting without any limitations. However, many in the general population undertake exercise not only so they can move freely but also so they can be strong, lean and balanced. This is their 'practical use', and it is therefore what functional training means to most people. (There are, of course, exceptions to this, particularly in programs for athletes and those with special needs.)

But how much of the functional training that you see around the place fits this description? Frankly, we have seen a lot of misuse of the term 'functional' in our time. People are undertaking the craziest exercises they can think of in the name of functional training. They are misusing popular tools such as kettlebells, ropes and rings, yet defining their programs as functional classes. But who are these classes and exercises functional for? What is their purpose?

The problem of dysfunctional 'functional training'

We have been in the fitness industry for a long period of time as trainers, presenters and gym owners. We have presented to thousands of trainers in over thirty cities and sixteen countries, and we keep encountering the same scenario: dysfunctional training.

Trainers are not assessing their clients thoroughly (or sometimes not at all), exercise selection is haphazard at best and there is next to no actual coaching.

---

1   Mel Siff, 'Functional training revisited', *Strength and Conditioning Journal*, vol.24, no. 5, 2002, pp.42–46.

MINIMAL SCREENING

First, the lack of assessment.

In 2013, we travelled in the US for self-development and to visit some well-established gyms. We attended one gym that had an amazing culture and energy. The trainer was likeable and very knowledgeable in many ways. We joined his afternoon class: a 'workout of the day' (WOD) that every client was doing that day. It was made up of rounds of snatches and sprints. We had to complete twenty barbell snatches and a 400-metre sprint, five times through.

We regard the barbell snatch as a high skill-level exercise. You need great mobility through the hips, shoulders and thoracic spine to execute it well. It is a power-based movement and demands excellent neuromuscular coordination. The right to perform this lift should be 'earned' through dedicated and carefully progressed movement training. Yet, even though we were two people the coach didn't know from a bar of soap, we were not screened. Instead, we were encouraged to lift heavy loads overhead dynamically for a high number of repetitions – with exhausting sprints in between!

We are both very experienced trainers and exercise at a high level on a regular basis. However, our trainer did not know this. He coached the snatch extremely well, but the lack of screening and programming was concerning. This programming methodology is a sure-fire way to encourage compromised technique and compensatory movement when training clients.

POOR COACHING

Alongside this lack of proper client assessment, we've noticed a general lack of quality coaching.

A popular movement in the industry is 'smashing your client'. We used to train at one of Sydney's most famous beaches. Trainers frequent the beach in droves with groups both large and small. One day, we observed a trainer taking two clients through a session. One of the clients was very overweight and looked like a novice – he was probably in one of his first sessions. The trainer was barking orders at his charges in a loud and aggressive voice, ignoring the fact that this client was clearly tired, distressed and overwhelmed. In fact, this just seemed to inspire the trainer to yell louder and more aggressively. The client then became unwell and vomited furiously. Did the trainer show any empathy or sympathy? Quite the opposite. He paraded like a proud peacock and forced the client to keep training.

What is the likelihood that this overweight man continued with training after such an experience? We certainly never saw him again. This individual, who had the best intentions to get fit, healthy and 'functional', was likely turned off exercise for a long time to come.

Since when is making someone vomit in a session regarded as a medal of honour? Why is making it hard for clients to get off a toilet seat for a week worthy of praise? When did abrasions on the hands or bruised knees become the goals of exercise? Is this going to encourage people to exercise? What is functional about any of this?

On the less aggressive end, we also see plenty of disengaged coaching. We have observed trainers checking their phones and talking about their weekends while 'training' their clients. Merely standing around and counting reps is not coaching. Couldn't just anyone do that job?

HAPHAZARD EXERCISE SELECTION

In gyms all around the world, we have observed clients being instructed on seated machines, isolating muscles in unnatural movements while their trainer counts repetitions. This rarely serves the client well or gets them to their goal of being functional. Our modern lifestyles have us seated for most of our days – should we then be seating people for exercise? Many clients struggle with everyday movements, yet their trainers have them performing unnatural movements that serve little purpose.

Moving off the one-dimensional seated equipment and using bodyweight and free-weight tools is often a step in the right direction. Yet even here, haphazard exercise selection remains an issue. There seems to be a movement among fitness professionals that the crazier the exercise, the better. We have seen people completing barbell overhead squats on kettlebells, lifting weights standing on Swiss-balls and performing box jumps on a pile of Reebok step boxes. There is little regard for establishing a foundation or ensuring safety. The mindset is that if it looks cool then it's worth throwing in the mix.

Many people coming to exercise for the first time struggle to move their own bodyweight with great technique and without compensation. Sedentary newcomers can sometimes barely get out of a chair or off the floor without difficulty. Why then is it common practice to load these clients up with as much weight as possible and make them lift? We see trainers push their clients to lift maximal loads when they haven't yet established a bodyweight foundation.

We saw a trainer recently showcase his clients' deadlifts and their 'impressive personal bests' on social media. We couldn't help but cringe, as these clients were displaying horrific hinging technique and placing their lower backs under significant load. This trainer was proud of his clients' feats of strength, but his good intentions were putting their health at great risk.

Loading poor movement patterns is rife in the fitness industry. There is a difference between helping your client hit a benchmark at all costs and really caring for that client and their health. Too often these intentions get mixed up.

THE OUTCOME – INJURY

Injuries are a prominent outcome of many exercise programs, yet they are almost always preventable. They result from a number of factors including poor exercise selection, haphazard programming and minimal screening (both initial and ongoing). This is a blight on our profession.

The scenarios we've brought to you are not uncommon. 'Dysfunctional' functional training is at epidemic levels within the fitness community. This is how people get injured and turned off exercise, trainers and gyms.

We need to do better if we want more people exercising, maintaining their exercise programs and making gains in their movement, strength and fitness. Indeed, we have a responsibility to our clients and ourselves to be better. We want to hit this global obesity epidemic head on and we are in the best position as trainers to have a big impact.

CHALLENGING THE STATUS QUO

We have written this book out of a desire to raise awareness about true functional training and how it can be life changing for the coach and client alike.

With thirty years of combined industry experience, ten of those operating the Functional Training Institute (FTI), Dan and I (Tarek) have cultivated a system of functional training through experimentation and learning. We have worked with the best in the fitness field, continually striving to improve ourselves so we can better serve our community. Our passion started with an idea, which morphed into a vision and materialised in an adaptive system for understanding and applying functional training.

Our goal as coaches and educators is summed up in one powerful vision: **To maximise the impact of coaches globally.** This is the attitude we hope will rub off on those coaches who seek to improve their craft by building awareness of movement and a training approach that is fluid, dynamic and ultimately adaptable to the needs of the clients.

Accordingly, we want to give trainers and coaches a clear system to help them assess and screen methodically, build good movement foundations and coach with a passion, all with the aim of preventing injury and, ultimately, getting clients moving with purpose.

This has placed Dan and me, and indeed FTI, as a global leader in functional training, serving thousands of trainers and coaches with a vision to reach many more thousands to come.

It is our belief that we need to be training people so they move better, become stronger mentally and physically and are fitter and happier. We need to change the way we conduct our training sessions so we see more clients training – and training *for life* – because they have come to enjoy it and reap its fruits. Haphazard, dangerous, futile and negative training needs to stop; in its place, we need training that is purposeful and functional. The Adaptive Functional Training System is the answer.

Introducing the Adaptive Functional Training System

The Adaptive Functional Training System (or Adaptive FTS, as we often refer to it throughout this book) is a progressive movement system that can help a majority of people function optimally. These include mobilisations, releases and activations to undo our modern postures, alongside exercises based on primal patterns such as squatting, lunging, pulling, pushing, carrying and twisting to help people get lean, strong and balanced.

The word 'adaptive' is used with the intent to jolt the trainer and coach out of a rigid and one-dimensional approach to movement training. Without the presence of mind to be flexible and willing to 'change things up', we become complacent and lack the growth mindset required to find new solutions.

Another word we have used with purpose is 'system'. We firmly believe that without a clear system, functional training devolves into a guessing game. As we've discussed already, lack of assessment, random programming and poor coaching are the three dangers that this guessing game can bring. In this book, we want to shed light on the positive elements of functional training that can bring results to clients and success to the coach. These positive elements are aimed at promoting optimal movement in a progressed, flexible and easy to follow system.

Functional training usually involves a multitude of movements that lead to an enhanced and coordinated relationship between the nervous and muscular systems. The brain operates and controls movement based on motions, not individual muscles. It is the programming of a diverse set of movements that leads to enhanced output as the improvements in strength and coordination are transferred from one movement to another.

A majority of functional movements are multi-joint, and a good functional training program should incorporate movements in multiple planes. You will find that in the Adaptive FTS a majority of the exercises are performed standing, either bilaterally or unilaterally. Furthermore, exercises include multiple joints and cover the fascial and sling systems, and many cover all three planes of motion. However, some muscle groups require isolation to activate them for bigger movements. These movements serve a function as they enable us to undertake gross movements more efficiently. We've therefore included these as central to the Adaptive FTS.

Programs should always be personalised within this context and this is a key component of the system. Variety and fun are also an integral part of the functional training philosophy, as fleshed out in this book.

FTI Adaptive Functional Training System model

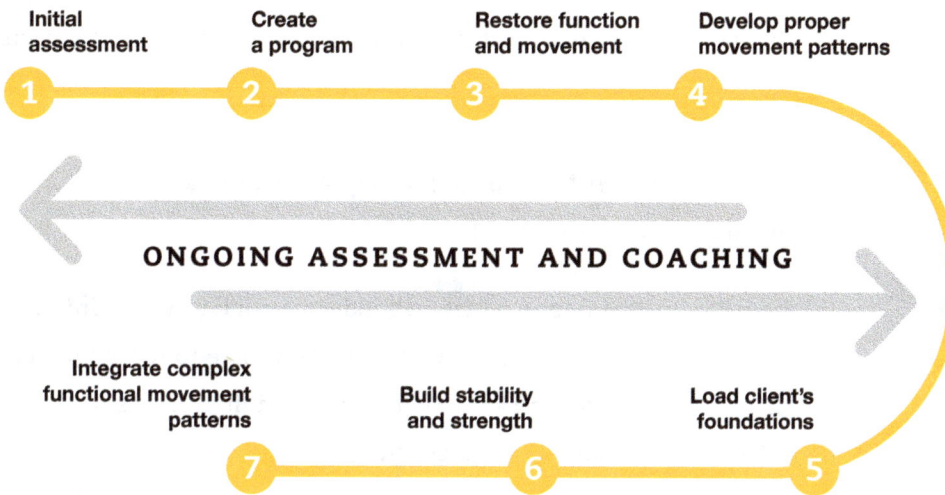

The Adaptive FTS strives to model excellence with systems and principles, but in a fluid and non-rigid way. Functional training from the perspective of a coach is not merely amassing a vast array of exercises; it is about how best to apply the functional 'tool' that will provide maximum benefits. These benefits are not only seen in physical gains or appearance, but also in the level of enjoyment and skills attained as the concepts, principles and philosophy of functional training are absorbed.

Here's an overview of how this book will guide you through the Adaptive FTS:

Part 1 – Coach with Purpose: The Art and Science of Coaching

The first step to becoming a leader in functional training is mastering the art and science of coaching.

This is a neglected aspect of training, often not given the level of importance it warrants. Coaching foundations addresses the big picture ideas like what makes a great coach (and how you can become one). We look at how to foster culture, connection and challenge (the three Cs) in your training approach, which all set the tone for purpose driven functional training. This will be supported with questionnaires and personality profiling to assist in implementing the three Cs in your own unique coaching philosophy. In coaching technique, we look at two vital aspects of coaching in action: cuing and feedback.

Part 2 – Assess with Purpose: Injury Awareness, Prevention and Monitoring

Whether you are training an athlete, a builder or your lovely grandmother, an assessment is a necessity. However, at FTI we like to recognise that assessment is not a once-off activity. There is the initial assessment, and then there's the ongoing assessment that should take place in any given session. What's more, both elements of assessment are integral to being an injury-aware and injury-preventing coach. The need to cultivate the 'coaches' eye' is an important ongoing feature in the pursuit of excellence and the evolution of trainer to coach.

Part 3 – Move with Purpose: The 5 Pillars of Functional Training

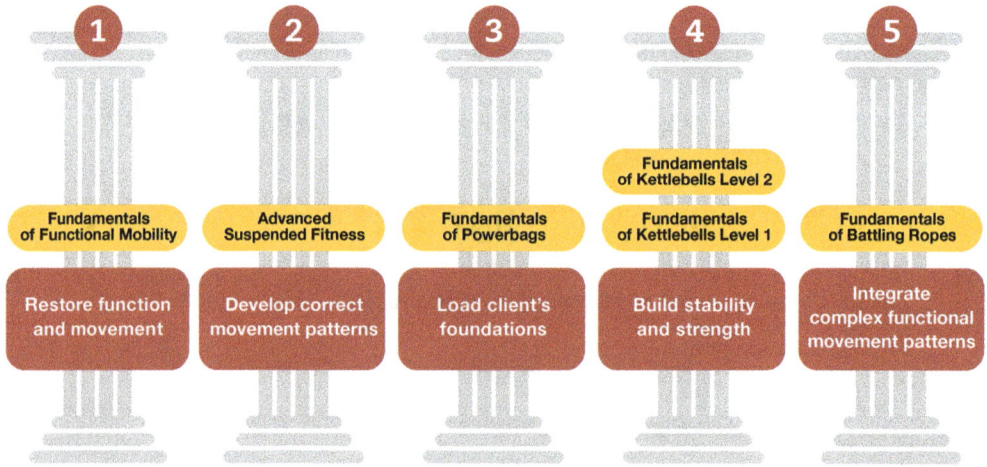

This section is the 'nitty gritty' of the application of functional training methods and is the foundation on which programming for functional training is built. We cover the five sections extensively. Each of these pillars, while understood initially as linear, allows the coach to then become more fluid and creative. This is seen when establishing the types of movements and the necessary progressions and regressions to safe, fun and ultimately successful programming. The five pillars are:

Pillar 1 – Restore function and movement

To perform a given task optimally, be it an overhead kettlebell press or a barbell deadlift, mobility plays an integral role. If we are to become, in the words of mobility guru Kelly Starrett, 'a supple leopard',[2] we need to integrate all of the following into our training:

- Joint preparation
- Mobilisations
- Activations
- Movement preparation
- Stretching

These are examined in detail in this pillar as we examine what best practice should look like for a trainer or coach entering the potentially murky space of function and movement restoration.

Pillar 2 – Develop proper movement patterns

Here we explore the primary movement patterns as we begin to build a foundation for optimal movement performance (whether in sport, training or life). As we like to say at FTI, 'If you can't do it, don't load it.' This especially applies to the client who has minimal functional training experience and those who have been sedentary for extended periods.

---

[2] Dr Kelly Starrett, *Becoming A Supple Leopard: The Ultimate Guide to Resolving Pain, Preventing Injury, and Optimizing Athletic Performance,* Auberry, Simon & Schuster, 2015.

The development of gross motor skills then becomes the focus for clients who need to learn to move more freely, which lays a foundation for coordinated and dynamic movements.

Our aim here is to develop these primary movement patterns with two methods:

- Suspension training
- Crawling-based movements

These are elemental to successful bodyweight programming and also provide the right base from which to start loading the client's foundation.

Pillar 3 – Load the foundations

Why load a client in the first place? The simplest and purest answer is for strength adaptations and the development of power. The success of a strength program depends upon learning the key lifts progressively and safely. This pillar focuses on the types of functional tools that will load a client in a non-intimidating, safe and progressive manner. We have selected the functional bag (sandbag/powerbag) as an example tool because it enables a client to perform loaded movements successfully via the movement patterns explored in the previous pillar.

Pillar 4 – Build strength and power

In this pillar, we advance from simply loading the foundations to building stability, strength and power. This should be at the heart of a good functional training program. Here we explore ways to make loaded movements more dynamic and progressive. As variety, progressions and regressions are a key ingredient in the use of functional tools, we focus in this pillar on the versatile kettlebell and how it can build stability, strength and power.

Pillar 5 – Integrate complex movement patterns

The final pillar is all about complex movement patterns. The incorporation of these complex movements into training develops neuromuscular coordination and enhances power for the client. This engages both anaerobic and aerobic systems, while simultaneously challenging the stabilising muscles of the core region. The focus tool for this pillar is the battling rope, although we also showcase complexes with other tools to add a greater degree of challenge for the client.

Part 4 – Program with Purpose: Bringing It All Together

It's time to let go of haphazard programming that adopts a 'one size fits all' attitude and does not take into account all the progressions, regressions and variations that will work best for a client. Our programming approach is the antithesis of this philosophy.

First, we cover programming theory in depth. We look into progressive and structured programming methods with solid principles. We show you how to use the 5 Pillars within a flexible periodisation model that will work for a variety of client styles, goals and fitness levels.

We also provide you with a sample program to get you started. One of the most critical and arduous programming tasks is creating a catalogue of functional exercises with the necessary progressions, regressions and variations. In our programming continuum platform, we have done just that and provided you with a blueprint for structuring classes and sessions that will also maintain the characteristics of a fluid and adaptive program.

Who is this book for?

You may be a seasoned trainer with years of industry experience, a new trainer off the block or an aspiring trainer. Perhaps you are simply a fitness enthusiast who wants to know more about functional training. Whichever cap fits you best, if you are curious about functional training and want to understand the positive changes it can bring, then this book can channel that curiosity into a meaningful and worthwhile pursuit.

Whether you are looking to improve upon your existing knowledge, better incorporate functional training into your business or simply enjoy the multifaceted benefits of functional training for your own health and fitness, then this book is the solution.

It is our great wish and hope that this book will play a significant part in your movement journey and provide a framework for your future success.

Part 1: Coach with Purpose

The Art and Science of Coaching

Coaching Foundations: The 3 Cs

'A trainer lights a fire under someone.
A coach lights a fire inside of someone.' – **Martin Rooney**

The true impact of a coach can be seen in how well he or she sets up the client for success. The quote by the great Martin Rooney from *Training for Warriors* captures this point well. Are you empowering your client to take it upon themselves to perform an exercise regimen on their own? Have you provided enough autonomy and variation in your sessions or are you dictating and controlling every single minute of workout time?

We have spoken to hundreds of coaches who have undertaken our technical and business programs. A common theme among them is a reliance on what's new and fashionable in the industry and a move away from the fundamentals. But looking for something new or following a wider trend is not the way to ignite that internal spark in clients. Good coaching is less about the gadgets you use and more about the way you are connecting with your client.

A few years ago, one of my coaches made each of his sessions memorable, not just by providing state-of-the-art equipment and a dazzling program, but through the way he connected, personalised the session and made it meaningful. This is what made him stand out: he cared, he was present throughout and he brought a sense of purpose to everything we did. One example is how he taught me to bring awareness to my breath as I moved through various sequences. This made every movement matter, to a point where I really began to feel the benefits of every subtle movement.

To be coaches, not just trainers, we need to have strategies in place to educate and enhance our clients' sense of possibility. Have we instilled a vision of mastery they can aspire to? Are we having an impact on our clients outside of sessions? Technical coaching and delivering programs are a very important part of the coaching process, yet they are not going to light that fire that will have our clients enjoying movement and exercise regimens when they are not under our guidance. How can we make our coaching more purposeful to a point where our clients rave about it and crave movement?

You will know that you have the right coaching foundations in place when your clients start to become 'raving fans'. In his book on this subject, Ken Blanchard describes a raving fan as 'a customer who is so devoted to your products and services that they wouldn't dream of taking their business elsewhere and will sing from the rooftops about just how good you are'.[3]

You'll find many raving fans attached to established businesses like Virgin and Apple, which have created cultures that lead to member retention and captivated clients. What can we learn from these successful entities?

Since we are talking about fitness, let's look at an example from our own industry.

One of the biggest and most successful fitness brands of the past ten years is CrossFit. Now, CrossFit is often considered controversial within fitness circles due to high rates of injuries and poor programming. But let's be a little more open-minded about where CrossFit has truly succeeded, and that is in creating raving fans. They have created a true symbol of 'cultural elitism' that revolves around hard-core fitness, paleo eating and a clean lifestyle.

---

3   Ken Blanchard, *Raving Fans: A Revolutionary Approach to Customer Service*, New York, HarperCollinsBusiness, 1998.

The allure of aspiring to complete tough workouts and difficult exercises is enhanced by the culture of the 'box', which is what CrossFit calls its gymnasium. Workouts are often splashed on a whiteboard and members are given targets to hit. Meanwhile, the internal environment of the box is conducive to member interaction, and participants bond around the elitism within the community. In other words, CrossFit has created a culture that is aspiration and comradeship rolled into one.

Having 'raving fans' brings benefits for you as coach. Clients who are happy with your service will not only stick around longer but will tell others about your good work and the impact you are having on them. This is not just beneficial to the coach; it's also beneficial to the client, who feels that they are a part of something special and begin to see results.

In this chapter, we want to look at the foundations that will help you evolve from an adequate trainer to a coach with purpose, creating raving fans in the process. We do this by introducing the concept of the 3 Cs, which stand for *culture*, *connection* and *challenge*.

The 3 Cs

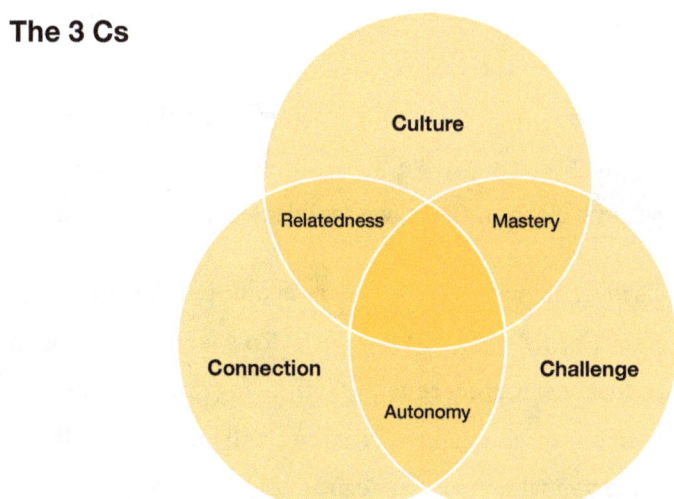

Each of these Cs forms an integral part of what defines you as a coach and makes you stand apart as a leader in your field.

Culture

The first 'C' is culture, and it's the foundational element that needs to be in place before all else.

When I (Tarek) opened up Primal NRG Fitness in Sydney with my business partner at the time, Ray, we spent many hours discussing what we wanted from this venture. We didn't want simply another gym; we wanted a special place where members could connect, train and become part of a culture that was making a clear difference – to each member but also the community at large. We wanted to cultivate an environment where clients became friends, encouraged one another and looked forward to each training session together.

Establishing a culture that will create raving fans out of your clients is an art form. It requires you to clearly define a philosophy, create a set of core values and identify a lasting vision. Without these, culture becomes just another interesting idea.

In our early days at FTI, Dan and I did not have a defined philosophy, vision or set of values. Even though we were living them out, it was not until we wrote them down and had our team contribute their thoughts that we became clear about what we were doing and where we were going. Once we became clear on these, we really started to go places.

The process of discovering what you stand for is a unique undertaking. What is it that makes you stand out as a coach? This is not about being better than other coaches; it is more to do with being grounded in who you are. The act of defining your vision and values will provide the clarity and direction to take you wherever you desire.

But giving your clients a sense of purpose needs to come from a deeper place of purpose – your own. Simon Sinek has popularised the importance of establishing your 'why' in his famous book *Start with Why*.[4] Before launching straight into a set of values or a vision statement for your business, you'll benefit from having a clear sense of what's driving *you*.

To help you get started, grab a pen and paper and answer the following questions:

- What do you stand against (as a coach)?
- What do you stand for (as a coach)?
- Why did you enter the field of coaching?
- Who were the people along your path who made a lasting impact on your journey?
- Where do you see yourself in ten years' time?
- List five things you are most passionate about in coaching.
- List three to five strengths you possess (for example: hard worker, intuitive, problem solver).

Your answers to these preliminary questions will likely provide you with enough sense of your 'why' to help you create a unique culture in your own coaching practice.

Now you're ready to define the philosophy, values and vision that will support your 'why'.

PHILOSOPHY

A philosophy is, by definition, a theory or attitude that acts as a guiding principle for behaviour.

In other words, your philosophy is how you convey your beliefs in a concise and real way to your clients. It is intrinsically linked to your values, but is not the same thing. Nor is it the same as your 'why', although it should be

---

[4] Simon Sinek, *Start with Why*, New York, Penguin, 2009. To understand Simon Sinek's message in a nutshell, watch his TED talk: The Golden Circle' Clip, https://www.youtube.com/watch?v=I5TwOPGcyN0

heavily informed by it. Instead, you could think of your philosophy as a summary of what you stand for and live by, applied to your coaching. For example, the functional training box Primal NRG Fitness has summed up its philosophy in three words: *Results, Progress and Community*.

So, how do we go about defining our philosophy?

First, create a philosophy statement for yourself. Having your philosophy summed up in a few words or a sentence, which appears on all your social media streams, marketing, clothing and your gym/box, is another step to take. It's good to keep things simple. You don't need to lose your way in complex terms or definitions, which can be off-putting or daunting for clients. In keeping it simple, you will come across to your potential and existing clients as the trustworthy professional you aspire to be.

Second, capture that statement in visual form. One of the most powerful ways to achieve this is via branding. Creating a symbol or logo that captures who you are paints a thousand words and more.

Your philosophy should be powerful enough that when someone asks you what you do, you can tell them about yourself and what you stand for with confidence. You want to influence and win them over with your passion for what you do and what you stand for.

EXERCISE

Write a paragraph (no more) on what you do and why you do it. Include:

- **Your unique training style (the technical)**
- **Your unique positioning as a business (your culture and niche)**

Revise your paragraph and highlight the key words from this.
Then condense your philosophy into a few words or a sentence.

Your philosophy then becomes part of your selling point for acquiring new members/clients.

VALUES

The second great practice for culture creation is to establish your set of values. These are the core principles that make up how you operate as a coach, and they form the essence of your philosophical statement.

By defining what you stand for, both for your own sake and the sake of your clients, you are ultimately standing against anything that stands in opposition. You therefore only need to define yourself in positive terms, rather than negative. For example, when one of your key values is 'We strive for excellence in service and programming delivery,' you don't need to say, 'We stand against poor programming.'

At Functional Training Institute we have defined our values as:

- World-class in content, delivery and service
- Fostering collaboration to serve others
- Creating and revolutionising industry standards
- Solution focused – treating obstacles as opportunities in disguise
- Tenacity and persistence – facing challenges with grit and determination
- Pursuing excellence – striving for progress and not perfection
- Cultivating an environment of empowering others through education

8 Core values to achieve our vision

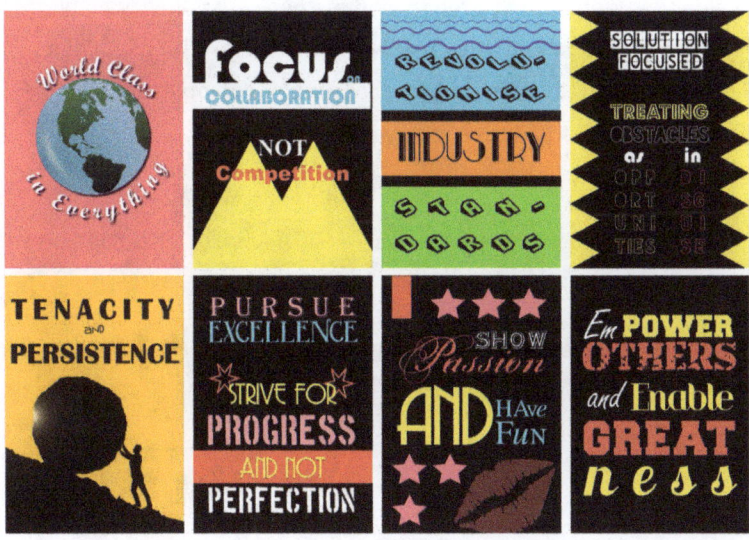

In the process of writing our values, we involved our key team members, office support team and presenting faculty to help determine what constituted our values at FTI. We encourage you to take up the same process.

As a whole, FTI has operated on another plane since crafting our values. This is only possible because we live and breathe them on a daily basis. To give a working purpose to our values, every week our team conducts a meeting in which we refer to a specific value that each team member has seen in themselves or in another team member. The amount of positive energy and productivity that this generates is staggering.

We have also displayed our values and vision in all our education content so that course attendees get a sense of who we are and what we stand for. It makes us accountable to those values and keeps us focused on how to best serve our community.

EXERCISE

Write out a set of values that you stand for. These can be personal, but for this exercise should have application in your professional setting. For example: hard-working, punctual, empathetic, collaborative, solution focused.

To do this, you may want to find a list of values (there are many available on the Web) and circle ten to twenty words that resonate with you. Then narrow this list down to the most relevant for your coaching. I suggest making your set of values no larger than eight.

Once you have selected your values, write a sentence or paragraph explaining what this value is, why it is at the core of what you do and how it is best reflected in you.

You can then use your unique set of values when hiring your team members to ensure you get the right people on board.

VISION

What do you do and how do you want to be viewed by others? What is the best you can be and how can you deliver your 'why'?

Your vision statement is a lasting statement that guides the business for the long term. It must reflect the company's culture (see philosophy) and what it stands for (values). Keep it short and succinct and make sure it matches up with your philosophy and values.

Here's a wonderful example of a complete vision statement:

'Our vision is to be Earth's most customer centric company; to build a place where people can come to find and discover anything they may want to buy online.' – Amazon

At FTI, our vision is short and to the point: *'To maximise the impact of coaches globally.'*

Your vision needs to be communicated. It should be splashed across all your mediums: Facebook, your website, brochures, merchandise and anywhere else.

If you don't have a vision statement, now is the time to think through what your vision is. Whether long or short, it should flow out of your values and be authentic to you.

EXERCISE

To get the ideas flowing for your vision, consider the following questions:

- **What problems do your clients have that you can solve?**
- **What outcomes would you like your business to achieve for people? For yourself?**
- **What words describe the experience you want clients, customers or members to have when interacting with you/your business?**

Once you have thought these through, have a go at writing out a statement that captures your ideas. This can be long, like Amazon's vision statement, or shorter like FTI's version. Don't worry if it's not perfect: this can be your 'working vision', which will help inform everything else you do.

DEVELOPING YOUR CULTURE

When drawing all of these things together to create your unique culture, you'll want to think about how your philosophy, values and vision are applied both inside your gym or training space and outside it.

Our physical environment needs to have the right ambience, good and safe equipment and quality amenities. But the biggest environmental influence is not the physical set-up, the equipment or the location of your gym, studio or park – important though these can be. As the coach, it is *you* who dictates the environment, much the same way a conductor commands her orchestra.

Much of the culture will be set by your own leadership. How will you be a diligent manager and an inspirational leader to your team? Oftentimes we can get caught up in the former, becoming a dictator that no one really likes. When you operate as an influencer rather than an authority figure, lighting that spark within others, you inspire your team members as well as your clients. All coaches and team members need to feel like they belong to the box, to a point where they feel it is as much their box as it is yours.

If you have a team or colleagues, then the culture of your box is a shared responsibility. Once you have the right people on board and they have bought into what you are about, they can then proceed to affect the culture within the box. They become the face of your business as much as you are. The idea is to be working in harmony under the same vision to such an extent that even when you are not there you really are not missed. I would exhort that this be the ultimate goal of a successful business. Your members will be drawn to the way your coaches interact with members on multiple levels.

Presence

Culture starts with the small things. It is the compounding effect of those small things that amounts to something significant. The culture of your box will be established from the way each member is greeted or welcomed to a class, through to the way they are farewelled at the end. A lasting impression is vital for a client, who will feel like a valued member of the community when you address her by name. Yes, remembering names is key to making a lasting impression!

Being present starts at the beginning of a session. If you are not there to greet your client and get a snapshot of their life leading up to the session, you have lost valuable information that could affect the day's training.

It is easy to be distracted and find your mind wandering during a personal training session. It will happen from time to time when you're tired or distracted by other matters. As long as you're aware and make an effort to re-engage, this momentary lapse in concentration does not need to ruin a training session. Far worse than poor concentration, however, is the habit of moving attention away from a client to check yourself in the mirror or check the latest Facebook status. Sadly, I've seen it happen!

Being present goes deeper than avoiding internal and external distractions. It is more about being engaged with your client for the entire session rather than merely being a passenger. A coach should be an active encourager, whether through silent presence or vocal support. A good coach will observe, encourage, correct and adjust to the needs of a client.

If you as a coach are not actively present during the session, then it is hard to meet the needs of a client – simply because you are not paying attention to what the client is telling you. You will not be enhancing your client's skills or fitness through proper coaching technique (see next chapter). What's more, you will not be observing them well for movement and injury screening or reading the physiological signs of the client, such as noticing whether they are stressed or tired coming into the session.

Here are the top five killers of presence:

- Not greeting client by name
- Mobile phone distraction
- Talking to other people during sessions
- Paying attention to oneself in the mirror
- Standing still and silent for the entire session

ONLINE RESOURCE: Watch the video we have created to highlight these points – http://functionaltraininginstitute.com/book-resources/

Relatedness

Relatedness refers to the universal need to interact with, care for and connect with others. It will be who is with us when and where we change.

Relatedness is one of the defining features of CrossFit's culture. They understand relatedness better than anyone in the fitness industry. It is little wonder that the number of CrossFit participants, boxes and communities has grown immensely over a short period.

Relatedness can easily be fostered within the training environment as well as outside it. Here are some of the ways you can encourage relatedness:

- Prioritise space in sessions to talk and interact (client to coach and client to client).
- Provide social events to encourage community growth.
- Create opportunities for clients to reach PBs as well as opportunities to celebrate them.
- Maintain regular contact with clients outside of sessions.

In this age of social media, there are many ways to develop client interactions and a sense of membership beyond the box. At FTI Global, we have found Facebook channels fantastic for keeping up momentum with clients outside of training sessions. Our business page on Facebook allows us to share content to the wider community and interact with other like-minded individuals and businesses. Meanwhile, our Facebook closed groups have provided added value, increased member interaction and fostered a sense of healthy exclusivity. Coaches and members share photos, videos and ideas, all of which help to foster great community. And of course, social events organised by keen clients are always a winner for building that out-of-session sense of camaraderie.

In all of these ways you impact your clients outside of the session, achieving a level of motivation and accountability not by way of control but through the sense of excitement grounded in your community and culture. The culture you have defined will spread like wildfire outside of your sessions, keeping clients motivated to stay on track and on the way to becoming raving fans.

Connection

Our second 'C' is connection. Now, connection can mean social and group connection, which is largely fostered by the culture you create. Here, though, we want to focus on the coach-to-client connection, which is fundamental to good coaching. The first element that forges connection is trust. The second is personalisation.

TRUST

The coach-client relationship cannot be founded on an egocentric approach. Roy Sugarman puts it profoundly and accurately:

'A client-centred focus is epitomized by listening, not telling. A client-centred approach increases a sense of trust that the coach is there for the client, as all parents should be for those they are charged with growing and supporting unconditionally.'[5]

---

5   Roy Sugarman, *Client Centered Training: A Trainer and Coach's Guide to Motivating Clients*, PTA Global, 2014, p. 67.

Before commencing any training program, your aim should be to establish the goals, history and profile of your client as a means of understanding their needs. When you do this, you are establishing trust. This trust should be re-established in the meet-and-greet stage before any individual session.

Trust is the lifeblood of any personal training or coaching business. It begins with the small things. The saying 'first impressions last' must be taken seriously. Presenting yourself professionally, making good eye contact and relating with warmth are all good starting points for establishing the initial trust that will encourage the client to show up next time. But if you keep making and breaking 'little promises' to clients, showing up late to their sessions or failing to make programming tweaks and variations for their specific needs, your training relationship will disintegrate. The bottom line is that a good connection keeps both you and your client engaged in the training process. This is not to be mistaken with keeping a client on your books to keep the business ticking over.

The job of a coach is to understand the client's expectations. This understanding needs to begin from the initial assessment phase (see Part 2, *Assess with Purpose*) and continue throughout the ongoing assessment and coaching of the client. The more you understand and treat your client as an individual, the clearer you will become about their expectations and needs. That's why 'personalisation' goes hand in hand with trust.

PERSONALISATION

Coaches, teachers and mentors in all areas of life need a basic understanding of how different people work so that you can personalise your coaching interactions.

At FTI, our focus is on making the training session dynamic, fun, challenging and adaptive. Being adaptive is partly to do with your experience as a coach, and partly to do with your attitude toward your client.

Tailoring your training sessions to each individual's needs requires some understanding of different personalities and preferred learning styles, which then enables you to communicate with each client uniquely and in a way that will deliver. This is the essence of being client-centred.

There are many different types of personality profiling out there that we can draw on. One of the more popular ones is the DISC Profile.[6]

Dr William Marston was one of the many psychologists and scientists who have tried to explore behavioural patterns. In 1928, following the completion of his doctorate at Harvard University, he wrote *The Emotions of Normal People*. Marston theorised that people are motivated by intrinsic drives that direct behavioural patterns.

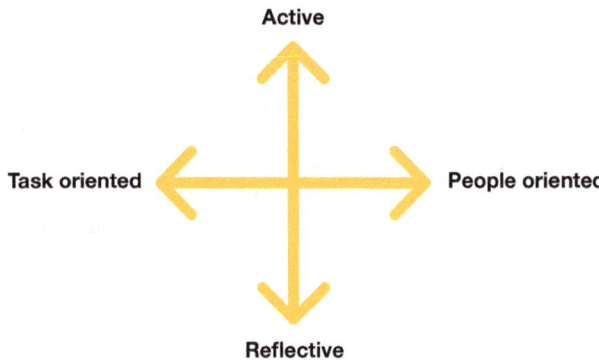

He used four descriptive characteristics for behavioural tendencies, which are represented by four letters of the alphabet:

D – Dominance
I – Influence
S – Steadiness
C – Conscientiousness

---

6   For a good summary of DISC, see A Rohm *A Powerful Way to Understand People Using the DISC Concept*, 2013, retrieved from www.discoveryreport.com/downloads/understanding-people-disc-personality-traits.pdf

The model is based on two foundational observations of personality traits in general behaviour:

- The internal motor or pace
    a) Active
    b) Reflective

- The external focus or priority
    a) Task oriented
    b) People oriented

We have all four of these traits, but one or two of them will dominate in us most of the time. Where a person's most dominant internal pace and external focus cross determines the type of personality they own.

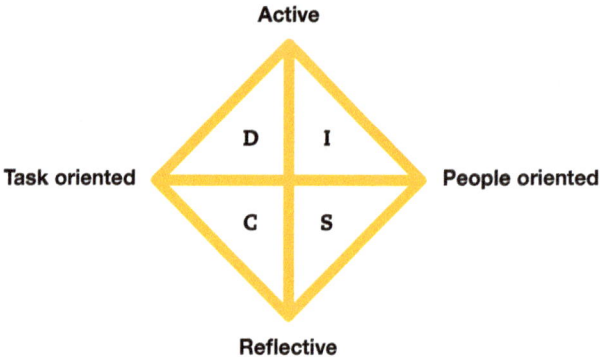

Active	+	Task oriented	=	Dominance
Active	+	People oriented	=	Influence
Reflective	+	People oriented	=	Steadiness
Reflective	+	Task oriented	=	Conscientiousness

The following table is a summary description of each of these four characteristics:

Style	D – Dominance	I – Influence
Characteristics	Focuses on getting things done, accomplishing tasks, and getting to the bottom line as quick as possible	Loves to interact, socialise and have fun Focuses on what others may think of him or her
Body language	Big gestures, leans forward, advancing	Expressive, friendly posture, amusing
Speech pattern	Directive tones, abrupt, interrupting, intentional	Talkative, varies tones, easily distracted
Key value	Respect and result	Admiration and recognition
Personality	Firm	Fun

Style	S – Steadiness	C – Conscientiousness
Characteristics	Enjoys healthy relationships, helping or supporting other people and working together as a team	Seeks value, consistency and quality information Focuses on being correct and accurate
Body language	Gentle gestures, reassuring	Unemotional, controlled gestures, assessing
Speech pattern	Conversational, warm tones, friendly, prefers listening	Unemotional, monotone, logical, focused, questioning
Key value	Friendliness and sincerity	Trust and integrity
Personality	Friendly	Factual

At FTI Global, coaches are encouraged to get educated about DISC so they are able to pick up the intrinsic drives of their clients and adapt their coaching.

The initial assessment is crucial to identifying the client's needs and wants. During this time, we probe the clients using the OARS method of motivational interviewing (Open questions, Affirmation, Reflective listening, Summary reflections).

Every question that we ask is open ended, to encourage the client to share as much information about themselves as possible and to give them a platform to basically open up. Throughout the interview, we also lead and pace the client by using questions like:

- What are some of your expectations from your training program?
- Why is reaching your goals important to you?
- In what ways do you believe that I can help you?

To bring us closer to understanding their styles, we ask questions like:

- Do you like to feel challenged or structured when you perform tasks?
- Are you a person who loves variety or prefers routine?

To ensure that the client feels safe talking to us and that we are listening to them attentively, we affirm their statements and provide reflective summaries of what they have said. This ultimately builds trust between the coach and the client.

All this is done while taking notes on phrases and words that they use. These notes allow us to gauge what kind of style we are dealing with and allow us to personalise the approach. By reflecting a client's goals and style back to them in their own words, we have created an environment that lets the client feel safe and comfortable. We are now speaking their language at their level.

This is an ever-evolving approach, and we build a clearer picture of the client's profile as we obtain ongoing feedback in every session.

This capacity for constant change and nuance in personalisation is what differentiates a mere trainer from a coach. The coach provides an enhanced fitness experience by making it all about the client on a subconscious level, interacting in the way he or she most wants to be communicated with.

Before implementing this in your own work, we strongly recommend that you first test yourself and understand what kind of personality *you* are. This will help you adapt your own communication styles to the client.

Here is a summary of how you can work with people of different styles:

Communicating with the D

Characteristic	Approach
Concerned with being the first	Show them new opportunities and how to win
Think logically	Display reasoning
Want facts and highlights	Provide concise data
Strive for results	Agree on goal and boundaries; support or get out of their way
Like personal choices	Allow them to 'do their things' within limit
Prefer to delegate	Look for opportunities to modify their workout focus
Want others to notice accomplishments	Let them take the lead, when appropriate, but give them parameters
Tendency toward conflict	If necessary, argue with conviction on points of disagreement, backed up with facts; don't argue on a 'personality' basis

Communicating with the I

Characteristic	Approach
Concerned with approval and appearances	Show them that you admire and like them
Seek enthusiastic people and situations	Behave optimistically and provide upbeat setting
Think emotionally	Support their feelings when possible
Want to know the general expectations	Avoid involved details, focus on the 'big picture'
Need involvement and people contact	Interact and participate with them
Like changes and innovations	Vary the routine; avoid requiring long-term repetition from them
Want others to notice them	Compliment them personally and often

Characteristic	Approach
Often need help getting organised	Do it together
Look for action and stimulation	Keep up fast and lively pace
Surround themselves with optimism	Support their ideas and don't poke holes in their dreams; show them your positive side
Want feedback that they 'look good'	Mention their accomplishment and progress, and your genuine appreciation

Communicating with the S

Characteristic	Approach
Concerned with stability	Show how your idea minimises risk
Think logically	Show reasoning
Want documentations and facts	Provide data and proof
Like personal involvement	Demonstrate your interest in them
Need to know step-by-step sequence	Provide outline and/or one-two-three instructions as you personally 'walk them through'
Want others to notice their patient perseverance	Compliment them for their steady follow-through
Avoid risks and changes	Give them personal assurances
Dislike conflict	Act non-aggressively, focus on common interest or needed support
Accommodate others	Allow them to provide service or support for others
Look for calmness and peace	Provide a relaxing, friendly atmosphere
Enjoy teamwork	Provide them with a cooperative group
Want sincere feedback that they're appreciated	Acknowledge their easy-going manner and helpful efforts, when appropriate

Communicating with the C

Characteristic	Approach
Concerned with aggressive approaches	Approach them in an indirect, non-threatening way
Think logically	Show reasoning
Seek data	Give data to them in writing
Need to know the process	Provide explanations and rationale
Utilise caution	Allow them to think, inquire and check before they make decisions
Prefer to do things themselves	When delegating, let them check procedures, and other progress and performance before they make decisions
Want others to notice their accuracy	Compliment them on their thoroughness and correctness when appropriate
Gravitate toward quality control	Let them assess and be involved in the process when possible
Avoid conflict	Tactfully ask for clarification and assistance you may need
Need to be right	Allow them time to find the best or 'correct' answer, within available limits
Like to contemplate	Tell them 'why' and 'how'

Learning to read your client's body language and asking them the right questions will unlock opportunities for you to adapt each session according to their needs. Knowing someone's personality type also helps you to understand how to communicate effectively with them and work alongside them toward their goals. Rather than telling the client what to do, you will start working with them to find solutions to their needs. This is a truly personalised approach to coaching.

ONLINE RESOURCE: https://discprofile.com/what-is-disc/overview/

Challenge

Our third 'C', challenge, is about providing enough stimulation and purpose in coaching that the client becomes highly motivated and invested.

What exactly is motivation? Simply, motivation is why we do things. The forces that create drive and provide motivation are complex. They may be biological, social, emotional or cognitive. Our aim in this section is to simplify motivation so that coaches can better communicate and engage with their clients.

Motivation is one of the most common words in the fitness industry – and one of the most misunderstood. Our Facebook pages are full of trainers posting videos of incredible athletic feats, inspirational speeches by well-known identities and trainers yelling at their clients, all with the intention of stimulating motivation. We see posts promising cheat meals or idealised bodies as supposed rewards for sticking with training.

As a society, we have embraced the 'carrot and stick' approach, using external motivators (rewards and consequences) to try to influence behaviour. Extrinsic motivation is defined as undertaking action for an outcome that is separate from the activity itself. We encourage the behaviours we want from our clients (attendance at sessions, adherence to dietary plans and so on) with external rewards such as free sessions, cheat meals and new workout gear. These are the 'carrots' for listening to us and adhering to our 'expertise'. If clients fail to adhere to our advice then we punish them with harder sessions, restrictive diets and negative feedback. These are the 'sticks' we use when we see behaviour from a client we don't approve of.

So, are these methods effective? While they might motivate someone in the short term, they fall short of changing behaviour over the long term and are not aligned with best knowledge and practice. Rewards can be used as a means of motivation, but they should be unexpected and offered after a task is completed. This is very different from trying to motivate a behaviour by offering a reward. We need to shift from 'if-then' rewards – '*if* you train an extra twenty minutes this week, *then* you can have that cheesecake' – to 'now-that' rewards, which reward something after it's done. For example, if your client achieves attendance in 100 sessions or lifts a personal best, you can reward that.

Ultimately, we want to encourage intrinsic motivation. Intrinsic (or internal) motivation is defined as doing an activity because of its inherent satisfactions. When clients are internally motivated, they experience greater feelings of enjoyment, accomplishment and excitement. Internal motivation has been shown to enhance long-term exercise adherence more than any other form of motivation. It sustains passions, creativity and effort. If you can provide an environment that stimulates internal motivation in your clients, then the likelihood of clients training more regularly and for longer will increase.

Self-determination theory proposes that we have three innate needs – relatedness, competence and autonomy.[7] Dan Pink similarly outlines three core needs – purpose, autonomy and mastery – that, though not identical, overlap with those in self-determination theory.

ONLINE RESOURCE: Watch this great video from Dan Pink about 'Autonomy, Mastery & Purpose' – http://functionaltraininginstitute.com/book-resources/

At FTI, we see four components that come together to create our third C, challenge. These are purpose, competence, autonomy and flow, which together help your client experience the highest forms of motivation and engagement with an activity.

---

7   http://selfdeterminationtheory.org

PURPOSE

A client will become truly motived when they experience a sense of purpose and fulfilment in their training. In Japan this is known as 'ikigai'. *Iki* means 'life' and *gai* describes value or worth. Essentially, ikigai is the reason why you get up in the morning. Your clients want to experience ikigai in their training. And this purpose needs to be about your *client's* needs, not your own.

Purpose (fulfilment) – creating emotional connections

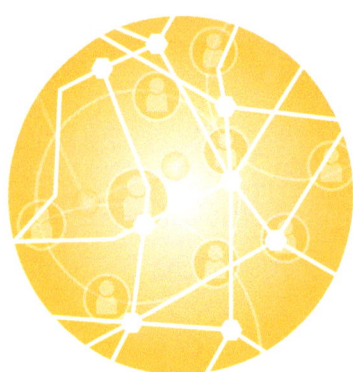

- **Purpose** equates to **Fulfilment**
- Without purpose your clients will make *little progress* and will *likely move on*
- Purpose is instilled by identifying the client's fitness and health links, desires and dreams – and then setting *realisting, accomplishable* expectations
- Coaching with purpose increases the *trust and connection* between you and your client(s).

As you can see, a strong culture and connection will go a long way to building your client's sense of purpose in training.

A sense of purpose needs to be infused into everything you set out to do:

- Purpose for the exercise or movement you give your client
- Purpose in the session you design
- Purpose in the program you create

You'll notice that every part of this book is about approaching functional training with a sense of purpose. You need to coach, assess, teach movement and program for your clients in ways that are meaningful to them and provide the ikigai they seek. If you don't have *client-centred* purpose at the forefront of your training system, your clients will stagnate in their training and lose their trust in you as a coach.

COMPETENCE

Competence or mastery is the self-perception that you can control an outcome. Feedback is absolutely essential in fostering your client's competence.

Quite often at our kettlebell courses we have a room full of people who don't believe they can perform a Turkish get-up. They see the exercise and believe it is too complicated. It is our job as educators and coaches to change the participant's perception and experience of their competence.

We do this by taking a complex and highly technical movement and breaking it down into much simpler phases. Their competence to perform the phases is high. We support this by giving each participant individual feedback on which elements they performed exceptionally well. We then bring the phases together and the participants perform the Turkish get-up with exceptional technique. Their competence to perform the movement is enhanced simply by focusing on the process or journey as distinct from the outcome or destination. By breaking the movement down into chunks and integrating coaching cues (which we will look at more in the next chapter), we make the process more worthwhile and realistic for them. This is key to creating engagement, enjoyment and mastery of new things such as a Turkish get-up.

Outcome goals have their place. When someone has a need to lose twenty kilos, the outcome is very important. We want the client to be accountable to this goal. However, getting the client to focus their attention on completing one session at a time and rewarding the process and habit formation itself builds the client's sense of competence and is far more motivating than a pure end-game focus. What's more, coach and client can enjoy the journey together.

AUTONOMY

Autonomy is the freedom to choose. People want to feel like they are making their own decisions and not being forced, either by other people directly or by external pressures. Perceived control is extremely important for happiness. We need to increase client autonomy in our training sessions by giving choices that empower them.

Autonomy begins at the start of the client-trainer relationship. Clients need to set their own training goals and not have them dictated by our preferences. We might have a functional training goal of completing a Turkish get-up with the beast (48 kg) because this is a huge feat of functional strength. However, this may mean absolutely nothing to a client whose goal is to exercise without feeling knee pain. We can guide our clients with their best interests at heart, but we need to be mindful that we do not enforce our ideals.

It is possible to expertly design and deliver an outstanding functional training program that gives autonomy to the client. With the Adaptive FTS, we do this through constructing a program and giving clients the choice of tool or exercise. For example, we will program a front squat, but the client has the choice of whether that front squat is with a powerbag, kettlebell or barbell. The level of choice could be even more general, where the client chooses the type of session. A client who exercises twice a week in our premises generally completes one strength session and one HIIT session. The client gets to choose the session type based on their energy levels and how they are feeling on the day. It is important to take a 'client knows best' approach in these situations.

There is a balance to strike between the coach as making the choice (control) and the client wanting to choose (autonomy). You may favour one type of exercise for your client over another, believing it provides a better outcome. However, if the client enjoys the slightly less 'effective' exercise the sacrifice is worth it when the payoff is an increase in autonomy and internal motivation.

The key to autonomy is clear, open and honest communication between you and your client. You need to know what they like and what they don't.

The best way to do this is to build regular program reviews into your training sessions. We are always asking the clients to rate the difficulty of a movement out of ten to measure their capabilities and competence. We also ask them how exercises feel and if they enjoy them.

ONLINE RESOURCE: To learn more about self-determination theory visit – http://functionaltraininginstitute.com/book-resources/

FLOW

The aim of any masterful coach is for their clients or athletes to experience 'flow' in their sessions. Flow is considered to be one of the highest levels of internal motivation one can experience. It is a state of complete immersion in which there is a perfect match between the perceived demands of an activity and the perceived abilities to meet those demands. When you bring together relatedness, competence and autonomy in your client's training, you have provided the right context for flow.

The level of challenge in an exercise, program or session shouldn't be too easy, nor should it be too difficult. Overly difficult exercises will diminish the client's competence. They will increase anxiety and have an adverse effect on the client's motivation. On the other side, if you do not provide adequate challenge then the client will become bored and disengaged. The effort to achieve the desired outcomes stretches the body and mind in such a way that the effort itself becomes the greatest reward. As a coach, you therefore need to consistently deliver exercises and programs that hit the sweet spot. Parts 2, 3 and 4 of this book will help you to strike the right balance between challenge and possibility for your client.

Creating an environment where your client is constantly seeking mastery in a particular exercise, skill or event is a great means of developing flow. I (Dan) experienced this with my kettlebell coach. Firstly, he had me set a meaningful goal in an event I enjoyed (autonomy). Secondly, he ensured this goal – an international certification in kettlebells – was extremely challenging yet achievable (competence). He then broke this down into micro-goals to help me achieve the outcome. Each session he programmed was a perfect balance between consolidation and new demand. I had to reach new levels of ability to achieve the goal. The outcome was the certification itself, which I gained, but the real joy was in the process of seeking mastery. I was constantly striving for perfection, although this could never be fully realised. Each session provided immense challenge and satisfaction at the same time, resulting in complete immersion in the training. I was in a state of flow.

Csikszentmihalyi, the founder of the Flow Model, has stated that flow is more likely to be met if a set of parameters is incorporated.[8] These are clear goals, clear feedback and skills that are congruent with the demands of the activity. Clear goals should be set by the client, have a timeline and be realistic. Clear and concise feedback tells the client how they are progressing toward their goals.

As coaches, we need to take heed of these parameters and incorporate them into our sessions. We have this immense opportunity to assist in the provision of flow taking place as we can manipulate the environment to reach the challenge-skills balance. Flow is harder to achieve in a sporting context because the challenge can be unpredictable. We can create a more definite level of challenge through programming appropriate movements.

Enjoyment of the training experience is paramount, as is an opportunity to use technical skills. This may include workouts where you incorporate technical lifts, such as the barbell clean, that have been learned over an extended period. The workout presents the client with the chance to showcase their newly found expertise. Less competitive situations can also generate more flow than highly competitive con-

---

8   An overview of the Flow Model can be found here: www.toolshero.com/psychology/personal-happiness/flow-model-csikszentmihalyi/

texts. Your client may experience more flow in a smaller class than in a big, competitive public run, for example.

Flow can be enhanced in a training session if you adequately prepare the client for what is to come. This might include communicating the session in advance. You also need to be equipped with coping strategies should your client find that flow is not being achieved. You may need to alter the feedback, task, challenge, goal and so on. The key is identifying the appropriate variable and making the change. The way a client feels after a training session can be an indicator of whether they experienced feelings of flow within the session. If the client is energised and revitalised, then this is a good indicator that flow has been realised.

A masterful coach knows their client in incredible detail. They can appropriately construct programs that achieve flow experiences. By balancing out their level of skill and matching it to a challenging enough program, states of flow can well be achieved.

Reflective questions

Can you recall when you achieved a state of flow? What were you doing? How do we get our clients to remain mindful when working out?

EXERCISE

Find an activity that is just challenging enough that you can perform it. Stick with it for 30–60 minutes. What did you experience?

Now think about ways in which you can encourage your clients to get into a state of flow. Design a program that is challenging enough for them to get into this state.

To become a purpose driven coach, you need to know yourself and what you stand for. Your philosophy, values and vision will help you define a strong and clear culture for your coaching business. The connection you make with these clients through being present, building trust and taking a personalised approach will lift your game from mere trainer to true coach. Through challenge, your clients will build the internal motivation to reach their goals. As you build on these foundations, your clients will become raving fans.

Now it's time to look at some of the technical aspects of coaching.

Coaching Technique: Cuing and Feedback

The craft of coaching lies in a commitment to continual improvement. A great coach commits to refining his or her level of instruction and adapting it to the needs of the client. Coaching instruction is the communication between the coach and client with the sole purpose of performing tasks as safely, efficiently and proficiently as possible.

When coaching, have you ever stopped to think, 'Is my client getting what I am saying?' I have. And it's easy to get frustrated at our clients for not 'getting it'. Yet the problem is more often than not due to our own lack of awareness rather than something in the client. Client struggle should be expected, and it is our job to learn to communicate the technique more effectively – or to create an environment that encourages them to figure it out themselves. I love the saying, 'The beauty is in the struggle.' For natural learning to take place, sometimes it is best to not interfere with the client getting to grips (pardon the pun) with their kettlebell swing or sandbag hold.

Coaching technique is not simply a matter of 'cheering on' our clients. It's about offering timely and meaningful cues and clear feedback that enables the client to develop their mastery and autonomy. Most of the work is done by close observation of the client as they perform something. The next step is to address where the movement dysfunction is, empowering the client not only to recognise and think about this dysfunction but to *feel* where they are falling short. The FTI coaching model of cuing and feedback offers a comprehensive way to elevate your level of coaching instruction.

Good instruction lies in the 'less is more' approach. Too much instruction can interfere with the natural learning process. Finding that sweet spot for what to say and when to say it is part of improving your coaching craft.

Cuing and feedback are subtle arts. It is one thing to be technically gifted as a trainer, but quite another to coach a client with purpose and lead them toward mastery. Great technique does not automatically translate into coaching ability. Nor does motivational speech and energetic delivery make up for a lack of clear instruction. The trainer who uses thoughtful cuing and feedback techniques to enhance the overall session experience for the client is the more skilled one.

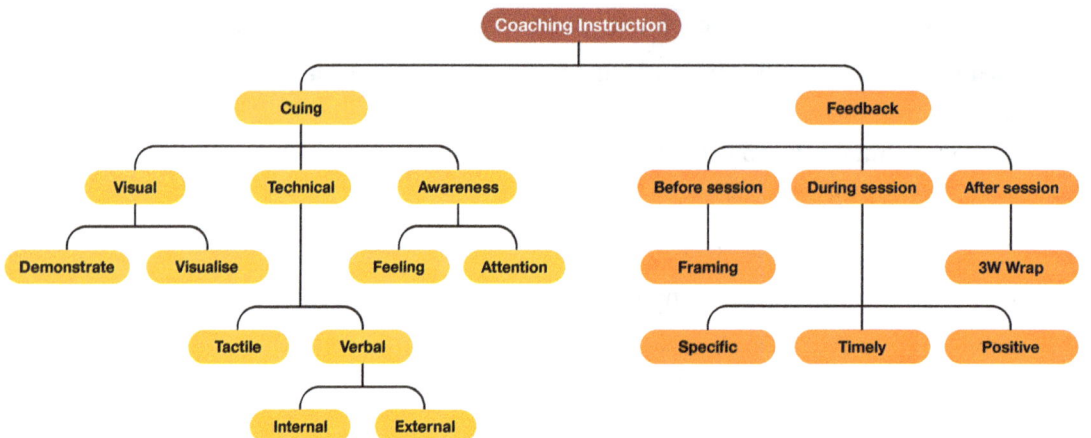

Cuing

At the Functional Training Institute, we incorporate a system of cuing to ensure that our trainers are coaching the client properly and personalising each session.

By becoming more intimate with and sensitive to how our clients respond, we can make complex movements and commands quite simple. Distinguishing between beginner and advanced clients and executing cues accordingly is essential. Adapting the demand of the movement and training session to the client or group takes skill and a deep understanding of the clients' needs.

WHAT ARE THE DIFFERENT STYLES OF CUING?

Traditionally, two methods of cuing have been recognised: visual cues and verbal cues.

In the flowchart that follows we can see a classic instructional analysis based on the visual and verbal methods of cuing clients. This has been examined with academic rigour by Dr Nick Winkleman, whose work has advanced our understanding of effective coaching based on the best methods of communicating to clients and athletes. Even though Winkleman's research and work has focused on athletes, the methods are effective for the general client population and their various needs and challenges.[9]

Effectively Integrating Cuing

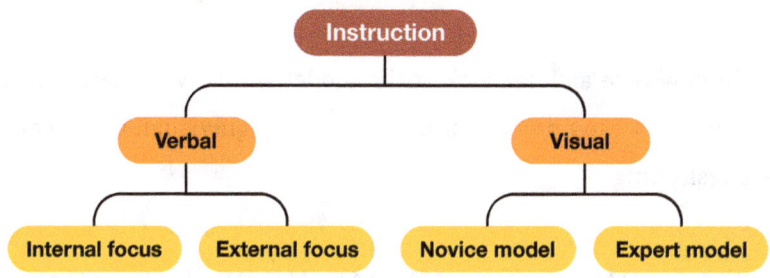

Great Coaches focus on verbal and visual cuing to:
- Manage (organisational coaching)
- Focus (ensuring the flow of the session)
- Adapt (adjusting to challenges) to the group's needs

A good coach will draw from a pool of teaching cues that will aid in communicating how best to teach a movement or exercise. As good as the verbal/visual model is, we have extended our coaching instruction to include an overlooked cuing skillset: tactile cuing and awareness.

---

9   https://www.otpbooks.com/coaching-movements-and-skills-with-nick-winkleman/

We feel that bringing in more kinaesthetic awareness to the cuing process is a necessary addition for general population clients.

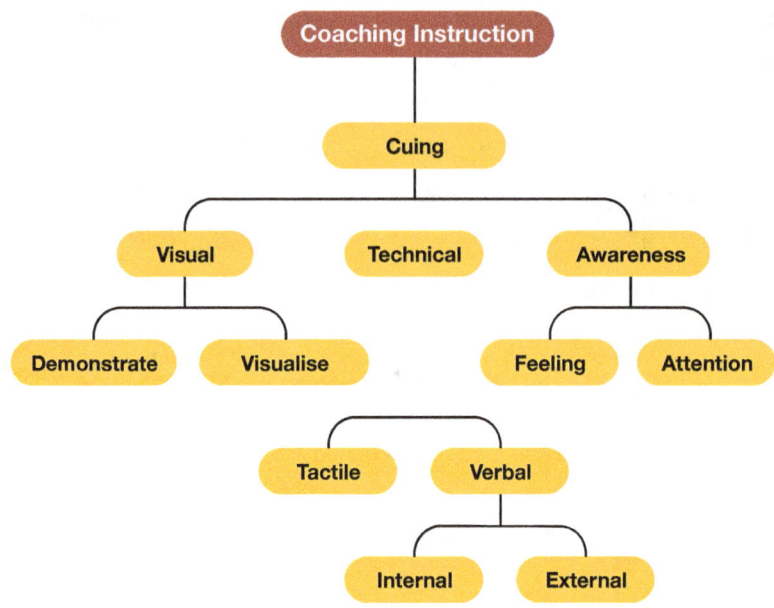

We will now take a closer look at the model and how we can influence the natural learning process of the client through visual, technical and awareness cuing.

VISUAL CUING (SHOW ME HOW IT'S DONE)

Visual cuing can be broken down into two parts: demonstrating the movement and visualising the movement.

Demonstrate

A majority of people – reportedly up to 70% of us – are visual learners. We see, and we do! Giving demonstrations alone will not suffice for teaching, progressing and reinforcing the key components that affect a movement or exercise. Nonetheless, the initial focus as a coach is to show how a movement or exercise is technically performed. For the kettlebell clean, for example, we will effectively perform the movement a few times first before breaking the movement down and uttering a verbal cue.

When demonstrating, ensure you orient each movement so that the client observes the movement from different angles and that nothing is missed. This promotes spatial learning. Getting clients to be aware of their surroundings (spatial awareness) is an imperative safety element of kettlebell or other functional training.

Visualise

Visualisation is a powerful way to improve quality of movement. Visualising is a skill that requires just as much practice as the physical side of performing the movement. Golfing great Jack Nicklaus used imagery to create focus and clarity in his golf swings. Here is what he remarked:

> I never hit a shot, not even in practice, without having a very sharp, in-focus picture of it in my head. It's like a color movie. First I 'see' the ball where I want it to finish, nice and white and sitting up high on the bright green grass. Then the scene quickly changes and I 'see' the ball going there: its path, trajectory, and shape, even its behavior on landing. Then there is sort of a fade-out, and the next scene shows me the kind of swing that will turn the images into reality.[10]

Why does imagery work? Because imagined events have an effect on the nervous system and mental processes similar to actual events. The brain can't tell the difference between vividly imagined events and the real thing.

Here is a little task that I (Tarek) have found to be very useful to integrate the demonstration and visualisation elements of 'show me how it's done' for clients.

---

10   Jack Nicklaus, *GolfDigest*, www.golfdigest.com/story/the-wisdom-of-jack.

- **Step 1:** Demonstrate the movement to the client – let's say it is a kettlebell swing.

- **Step 2:** Ask the client to visualise the movement, performing, say, ten mental reps. At this point you can aid the process by suggesting the image of a clock pendulum that's swinging from 5 to 9 o'clock as a visual descriptor. You can also add a rhythmic cue like 'tick-tock' for the timing of the movement.

- **Step 3:** Let them perform the movement with the kettlebell.

Keep in mind that using the verbal cuing component requires an understanding of what works and what doesn't for certain clients. Some will gravitate to visual cuing while others will respond better to verbal instruction. This is not a cookie-cutter approach.

TECHNICAL CUING – VERBAL AND TACTILE (TELL ME HOW TO DO IT AND HELP ME TO FEEL IT)

Technical cuing is comprised of both verbal and tactile instruction in the FTI coaching instruction chart.

Verbal

The audio learning style is powerful when used with visual instruction but needs to be used sparingly.

Coach Winkleman has a great saying: 'Attention is a limited resource capacity.' The more demand you place on your client via verbal commands, the less efficient they become. In my early days of being a personal trainer, I (Tarek) made the mistake of placing unrealistic expectations on my clients to perform a movement, only to be frustrated when they could not do it. It turns out that I was giving them too much verbal instruction, which interfered with their natural learning process. My approach at that point in time was that if I showed them a movement, I could then talk them through it and they would just get it. That was before I became intrigued with the coaching process and came to recognise that all people learn at a different pace and respond to instruction differently.

I can cue my client to perform a desired movement in a few ways. For example, when training for hip extension at the top of the kettlebell swing, I can say:

- Pop those hips
- Snap those hips

Via their neural feedback loop, your client will begin to associate a verbal cue with a visual execution. Remember, one step at a time along the pathway of progression. However, we can refine this further by using both internal and external cuing.

Internal cuing draws the client's attention to a local reference point, which is typically an anatomical reference point. It focuses attention on the muscles to affect a certain movement. A classic example is 'squeeze those glutes' as you come up from a deadlift.

Typically, most verbal cuing is done this way. Oftentimes there is an overload of instruction from coach to client, which means poor execution and confusion when performing a task.

That said, internal cuing plays an important role. With grind-based exercises such as a kettlebell row and other less complicated movement patterns, this form of cuing is still relevant for coaching clients. Here are a couple of examples we might use during a suspension training row:

- 'Pinch the shoulder blades together' – as when performing a kettlebell row.
- 'Keep the glutes lightly squeezed' – as when holding a plank.

We can also have an internal/external focus such as:

- 'Keep eyes fixed to the anchor point' – as when performing a battling rope wave. The external focus here is the anchor point and the internal is the eyes.
- 'Keep your elbows pointed toward the wall' – as when performing a double kettlebell press. The external focus here is the wall and the internal the elbows.

External cuing uses global references (the *training environment*) like the sky, ceiling or floor, alongside metaphors and analogies (the *training story*) such as 'pulling a cord' or 'exploding like a rocket', to simply and effectively communicate a technique to a client. In addition, there is a focus on the implement (the *training tool*) such as the kettlebell or whatever the client is using to perform a movement.

External cuing is useful for creating a focal point for more complex lifts or movements. Let's use the example of the barbell snatch. Arguably the most technical lift to perform in conventional training methods, the snatch requires timing and technical accomplishment and plenty of practice to master.

As coaches, we should deconstruct a movement like the snatch and get the client to practise it in parts so that the whole eventually becomes fluid and beautiful to behold.

In the final phase of the snatch the bar locks overhead, with the lifter coming underneath into a full overhead squat position (if performing a heavy and full repetition). Here are some external (global) verbal cues we can provide at different stages of the snatch:

- 'Explode the bar to the ceiling.'
- 'Look to the horizon as you drop under the bar.'

The external cues take away reference to anatomy (such as 'squeeze the glutes' or 'drive with the hips'). Dr Nick Winkleman has brought our attention to external cuing as a way to animate and contextualise a movement, harnessing the client's attention and directing it to the activity they are performing. In particular, when performing more complex lifts such as the snatch, there is an integration of multiple muscle groups and joints at play. To focus on one thing would be to the detriment of the movement. Secondly, from an instructional perspective, if we provide too much in the way of over cuing, in particular a focus on internal and singular muscle focus, then it will confuse the client's movement practice.

To take the process of 'cuing' to another level, we need to consider two fundamental building blocks that define 'external cuing'.

Animating the cue requires a deep understanding of movement patterns and the exercises that will be taught to the client. It requires that the coach has achieved a level of mastery specific to the exercise they are teaching their client.

By animating a cue, you are bringing a playful and visual means to getting a task done safely and efficiently for the client. The cue needs to be consistent and include a global reference point as previously mentioned. Rather than 'get the bar over your head', you include words like 'explode' and 'drive' to add meaning to the ultimate aim. To get the bar from the ground to overhead is a demanding task that requires speed and use of multiple joints, large muscles and global stabilisers.

But your client does not need to be bored with fancy anatomy and dull words. These words need to have an action emphasis (otherwise known as a verb or doing word), and should be spoken with the right tone in order to have full efficacy for the client. Try saying 'explode' in a low tone a few times. Now say it with a well-intended higher tone (but please do not scream, lest you scare your client silly).

Once you have selected appropriate action words, think of a reference point to complete the cue. Which of the following will spark more imagination and conviction in your client?

- 'Make sure the bar goes above your head' or
- 'Keep the ceiling from falling down'?

The latter verbal cue is global and uses creative and animate words: 'ceiling', 'falling', 'down'. It doesn't take an athlete to know that this point of reference relates to the overhead position. Although none of the technical terms are used, it will specifically encourage an overhead lock-out position in a jerk or snatch phase of a complex kettlebell or barbell lift.

Contextualising the cue is another way of employing external or global cuing to create a context that will act as a reference point for a client learning new skills, particularly higher-level skills such as a kettlebell high pull or snatch. One excellent verbal cue is 'pull the lawn mower cord'. For the weekend warriors who regularly mow the lawn, this reference point is perfect as it translates to the explosive drive phase of the snatch.

Contextualisation should be tailored to the individual where possible. If one of your clients is into fly-fishing, then that can be used to simulate the downward chopping movement when performing a cable row. Or if they are a golfer, then contextualise with the golfer's swing when performing the upward chopping movement in a cable row. Here's an example:

> **Aim:** To teach the client a dead kettlebell snatch.
>
> **Metaphor:** Imagine the kettlebell has a cord at the base, like a lawn mower cord, stuck to the ground. In order to bring the kettlebell into rack position, you need to powerfully 'yank' the kettlebell from the ground.

Some things to be mindful of when utilising this method:

- This is best adopted for one-on-one training as it is customised to the individual.
- You need to know the client's past history and current activities to know whether they will relate to specific actions such rock climbing, fishing or mowing.

- You need to stick with consistent terminology like 'throw the line' when performing a downward wood chop and relate the movement to that activity so it is cognitively embedded.

If my client doesn't know what a lawn mower is or is unfamiliar with the word 'yank', then it is simply pointless to try to convey it this way. This is why personalising the approach and understanding the preferences and styles of clients is important here.

Remember that verbal cuing is more than just barking an order to a client or group you are training. More genuinely and professionally, it is about communicating to that client or group how to best execute a given exercise or movement. This is done through a thoughtful analysis of the exercise being taught and breaking that movement down to achieve optimal results. Distilling a movement or an exercise to its purest and simplest form forces us to see it with a new set of eyes, to observe more and talk less. Let's call this the 'coach's eye'.

Not surprisingly, beginner clients often have a lower focus and can absorb less coaching instruction than more seasoned clients. Here is a series of steps useful when using verbal instruction for beginners:

- **Step 1:** Break down the movement, especially if it is more complex like a Turkish get-up with kettlebell.
- **Step 2:** Provide one cue at a time to help them become more adept at the movement. Less is more with verbal instruction.
- **Step 3:** Get them to perform no more than three to five repetitions over several sets.
- **Step 4:** Provide feedback after each set. This feedback should not alter their natural learning process.

A verbal cue is part of the purpose driven coach's arsenal. It will allow you to achieve best teaching practice, to keep the client engaged and, not least, to keep yourself present and switched on in the coaching session.

Touch

Touch is another integral part of learning, and this brings us to an often neglected part of a personal trainer's bag of cues. As you will see in our cuing flowchart, it sits alongside verbal cuing as a vital element of technical cuing.

By using tactile cues and props, we help to orient the client or group into a desired position in order to enhance proprioception (the ability to orient oneself in space). Proprioception underpins kettlebell – and indeed, all functional training – exercises.

You will come across clients who, after you have shown them an exercise and relevant progressions, just 'get it'. Meanwhile, others will struggle to come to grips with the show-and-tell aspect of coaching cues.

By sensibly cuing your client via touch, you can draw their attention to an area that they may ordinarily struggle to be aware of with visual and verbal cuing. For example, a touch of the upper traps in a kettlebell row, indicating to relax them, will give the immediate and specific sensory feedback that a verbal instruction cannot capture.

Obviously, touch needs to be safe and appropriate for the client. Some will be more comfortable with it than others, and the rare client may want to decline any physical contact. It is important to verbally indicate what you're intending, explain its purpose and ask consent when offering tactile cues. Above all, respect your client's wishes in this area.

ONLINE RESOURCE: To download the free Coach the Movement template, visit our resource link – http://functionaltraininginstitute.com/book-resources/

AWARENESS CUING (HELP ME BE PRESENT)

Sitting alongside visual and technical cuing is the skill of encouraging your client's awareness or 'mindfulness', which can be defined as 'paying attention in the present moment'.

There's been a flood of literature on the virtues of mindfulness training and its ability to enhance capacity for attention and awareness.[11] In the coaching context, our aim is to help a client grow in their kinaesthetic awareness: to have muscular sense perception (interoception) during a movement and be able to sense what their own body is doing while performing that movement.

Is 'paying attention' a limited resource capacity or can we increase our capacity to take more in? At any given time, we will encounter clients who have had a richer or poorer amount of attention during movement training. Couple this with their learning style and we come to realise we need to be customised and discerning in our coaching approach. A very powerful lesson I learned from my yoga coach many years ago was focusing my awareness on a particular part of my body that was tight. My coach would say, 'Breathe into the movement and focus your attention on your shoulders opening up,' in his calm and clear voice.

So, one way to faciliate kinaesthetic awareness is to draw a client's attention to their own breath. This gives them internal awareness in some similar ways to external touch. What my coach was teaching me was bringing my attention to what I was doing. Using my breath, coupled with his clear verbal instruction, I was able to go, as he would say, 'deeper into the movement'.

---

11   AP Jha, J Krompinger and MJ Baime, 'Mindfulness training modifies subsystems of attention', *Cognitive, Affective, & Behavioral Neuroscience* vol. 7 no. 2, 2007, pp. 109–19.

The main point I want to get across here is that *feeling* the movement from within is far superior to thinking through it. By helping clients perform a particular movement with awareness, you will not only increase their engagement but minimise their risk of injury.

So, in summary, use all of the following cuing methods to personalise your focus on the client and their movement quality:

Visual cues

- Show the movement first in different angles and multiple times.
- Break down the movement and teach that first, particularly for more complex lifts.
- Perform the progressions of the exercise.

Technical cues

- Select a meaningful word or phrase to accompany each phase of learning the movement or exercise. Less is more when it comes to verbal cues.
- Keep the cue consistent with a powerful projection of your voice as a coach.
- Use touch to cue movements when breaking down the exercise or when compensation or lack of activation occurs in the movement pattern.
- Use props to facilitate progression of a movement.

Awareness cues

- Integrate attention and feeling into movement practice.
- Get client to focus on the breath and a specific part of the body.

> **EXERCISE**
>
> **Come up with two external cues for the following exercises:**
>
> 1. **Barbell clean or kettlebell clean**
> 2. **Kettlebell swing or powerbag snatch**
>
> **Think of ways in which you can provide contextualised cuing for some of your individual clients. If you're not sure where to start, you may need to ask some clients about their preferred activities and hobbies, then think about how to incorporate ideas from their responses the next time you teach them a complex lift.**
>
> **Write down a list of internal cues for the following exercises:**
>
> 1. **Kettlebell row**
> 2. **Overhead press**

Feedback

Alongside cuing, integrating feedback – as long as it is the right type and the right amount at the right time – is another tool that marks out a purposeful coach from a mere trainer.

Once a client has been cued and coached in a movement and has performed it, a coach will usually offer feedback. Feedback refines the motor system 'by guiding the athlete toward a movement pattern in a manner that promotes implicit (self-correcting) processes'.[12] Each one of us possesses a natural learning process. We often call this 'second nature' because we have learned it to a point where we don't have to think about it. Timothy Gallwey, in his book *The Inner Game of Tennis*, refers to it as the innate learning mechanism.[13] However you want to describe it, the

---

12   RA Magill, 'The influence of augmented feedback on skill learning depends on characteristics of the skill and the learner', National Association for Physical Education in Higher Education, *Quest*, vol. 46, 2012, pp. 323–6.

13   W Timothy Gallwey, *The Inner Game of Tennis*, London, Pan Macmillan, 2015.

important thing to understand is that this inner learning process may be compromised with too much information overload.

At FTI Global, we aim to create a system for reliable feedback without overloading, or overriding, a client's implicit ability to self-correct.

In our feedback model, there are three important stages in creating a feedback loop that will keep your client engaged and enhance their experience of your sessions. They are feedback before, during and after a session.

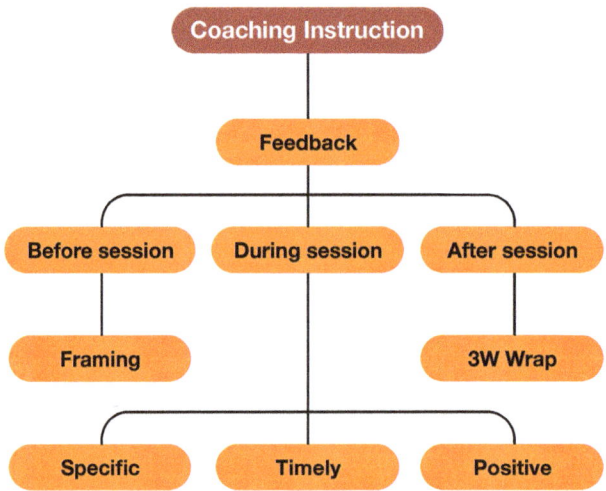

FEEBACK BEFORE A SESSION

It is easy to have the client rock up to your session and simply begin the workout. What is missed in this scenario is the opportunity to frame the session for the client. For example:

> 'Hi Tom, today we are going through an intense workout. We need to step up your training intensity as you are showing great gains to this point. We will be covering these movements ... let's first begin with this great warm-up. You got any questions? Cool, let's get started.'

Imagine if every session began like this. How would it affect your client's sense of purpose and autonomy? My guess is that it will absolutely skyrocket their engagement.

This level of feedback takes all but two minutes and also acts to clear up any confusion the client may have. Remember, tapping into the personality types here will add a further level of specificity to how you frame the session.

FEEDBACK DURING A SESSION

There are three distinguishing features to offering feedback during the session. Each one contributes to the success or failure of the session. In-session feedback should be specific , timely and positive.

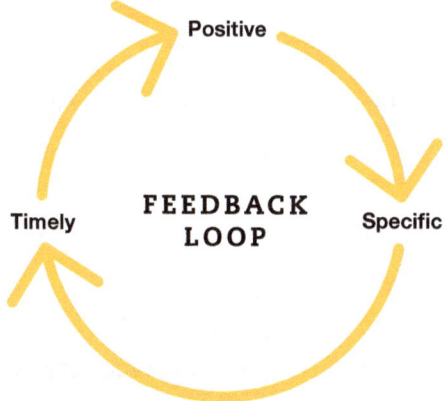

Specific feedback

Are you a coach or a cheerleader? If we are not present and involved enough in the session, it is easy for us to enter into what I call the 'drone zone', where you switch off and go on autopilot as your client performs their session. Have you ever experienced a session where the trainer was barking out instructions, occasionally offering 'good job, keep going' or other forms of empty feedback? I used to fall into this trap, but it is shallow and lacks the specificity that will help the client to competently perform the session. As tired as you may get, don't let yourself fall into a coaching lull like this.

To illustrate, here's an example: 'Your pivot on the bullwhip enabled you to perform the movement with a greater level of precision.' This level of specific feedback helps a client to home in on technique and understand its function within the exercise.

Good feedback requires a coach to have the presence and focus to offer precise and meaningful observations, whether this is through positive reinforcement and encouragement (positive feedback) or critique and correction (constructive feedback).

Positive feedback

Feedback during a session places most of the focus on process. When combined with positive comments about outcome, this can make for powerful feedback. In her great book *Mindset*, Carol Dweck refers to the process versus the outcome. The process is what leads to the mastery of something. Dweck therefore recommends acknowledging and praising a person's process as the best way to develop a growth mindset.[14]

In the context of our coaching, describing what your client has done and how this has contributed to improvement or mastery can help your clients to not only complete a session but also feel accomplished after a session. An example would be: 'Strong set! You performed an extra 5 kg on your front squat (specific feedback) with smooth technique (accomplishment).'

---

14 See interview with Carol Dweck, www.theatlantic.com/education/archive/2016/12/how-praise-became-a-consolation-prize/510845/

Feedback gone wrong

I (Tarek) recall a time many years ago when a coach on my team was providing negative feedback to one of his clients. Since this was a team training session, which this coach taught on a regular basis, it soon surfaced that one of our members was becoming unhappy with our gym, Primal NRG, and specifically that coach. What the member eventually reported to us was that she felt picked on, and the language of the coach was very negative, causing her to feel ashamed and belittled. This prompted me to act quickly to fix this major problem.

The lesson in all this was that the onus was on me, the owner, as the coach had clearly not properly integrated the methods of coaching we promoted at Primal NRG. Our gym prided itself not only on our progressive training techniques but on our vibrant and positive culture, including the way our coaches communicated and provided feedback to clients. From this failure, we revamped our systems and ensured a proper process, where coaches followed our methodology and provided feedback that was positive and specific.

Timely feedback

When coaching a client to perform a task such as a kettlebell press, we want to offer feedback, which is fair enough. However, the timing and content of that feedback is crucial.

Providing feedback during movement may impede the client's learning process. If you want to instruct as they move, provide one verbal or technical cue that will enhance and not deter their movement quality.

Feedback delivered during tasks can be distracting and take away from the implicit learning process, especially for beginners. As clients advance through your training programs, delivering feedback during an exercise will become useful as they become more proficient in processing the information. For beginners, adding a verbal cue that describes the movement such as 'push', 'pull', 'jump', may provide some measure of feedback that will help the client to be on task.

Feedback after the task is more helpful, particularly when timed and administered in a measured way. If you've taken the time to observe a full movement, exercise or set, you will be much more likely to provide the right insights that will keep them focused and engaged for the entire session.

The first step to providing appropriate post-task feedback is to observe impartially. If, as coaches, we observe without judgement, we can see the entire picture of how the client is performing in the sessions and even how they perform each of the movements. Once we become judgemental observers, we create a myopic coaching style that tends to zero in on one particular 'problem' as opposed to looking at the whole picture. But we need to be able to discern where an issue is coming from. Is it an ingrained dysfunctional movement pattern, a compensation for a niggly injury or simply a lack of focus? Have you broken down the movement sufficiently for them to perform it adequately? Is your program too difficult at this point in time? A coach who observes without judgement will take the time to weigh all the factors before speaking.

The second step is to ask the client for their own observations. Simple is often best, so ask them after a set, 'How did that feel?' or 'What did you notice in that last repetition?' Getting the client to describe their own experience taps into their implicit learning mechanism and deepens their own sense of intrinsic feedback.

The final step is to offer your observations about what is working well or not so well in a movement. If you can affirm their own feedback, do so, then give them something specific to take away. Consider the difference between saying, 'You got through the entire round without stopping – tremendous progress,' and something general like, 'You did well, but you can give me more?' Do you notice something negative about the second type of feedback? It is too general, and potentially damaging to the client's self-esteem, even though it is intended to make them aspire to greater things. Where your feedback can reflect their intrinsic experience, try to mirror that. If a client says their swing felt easier, you could say, 'Yes, your swing looked a lot more fluid and less forced than before.' When our feedback reflects a client's experience, they are empowered to learn the natural way and begin the process of mastery.

Quite often, we give far too much feedback and overwhelm our clients. At FTI, we see this in our courses when we get the trainers to coach one another. They give each other a thousand instructions on an exercise, then detail all the things that were wrong with it. More is not better when it comes to feedback. Commenting every time at the end of an exercise gets in the way of transfer of learning and may create feedback dependency. Asking the client questions is far more empowering than telling them how they looked or that their movement was not good enough. You want to draw the answers from the client and not give them your answers. Let's remember that a sense of competence and mastery increases the motivation levels of the client.

FEEDBACK AFTER A SESSION

This is often the forgotten piece of the feedback loop. At FTI, we encourage coaches to do what we call the '3 W Wrap'. The three Ws stand for 'What Went Well', but also for the three components of the wrap up, summarised as 'What, Why and When'.

> **What:** Recap the session and ask the client what they enjoyed about the session.
>
> **Why:** Provide feedback on what they did well and attach it to progress/mastery.
>
> **When:** Provide them with their training plan to work on and excite them about the next session.

The 3 W Wrap takes all of two minutes to do, yet this small investment of time ensures you finish off the session on a real high note. Consider it prep work for the next session and a way to increase the levels of motviation for the client. Within this form of feedback, the coach is tapping into autonomy (asking the client how the experience of the session was), mastery (what they did well and what their next focus is) and purpose (giving them a sense of achievement and fulfilment for getting through the session with intent and focus).

Conclusion

Being a purpose driven coach requires a model of coaching instruction that is based on solid coaching theory and principles. Every client is different, and understanding the difference between coaching a beginner and advanced client will shape the way you program.

As coaches, your words matter. The quality of instruction you give is seen directly in the quality of movement and progress your client gains. Without good coaching foundations and technique, the essence of good programming is lost. Having a model to provide the best cuing and feedback will ensure you have a foundation to design and deliver sessions with confidence, courage and professionalism.

Part 2: Assess with Purpose

Injury Awareness, Prevention and Monitoring

The Background Story on Fitness and Injuries

We are living at a point in time when profoundly sedentary people are being urged, for all manner of health and lifestyle reasons, to embrace fitness programs. People who are starting from the furthest behind physically are attempting to leapfrog ahead into being, looking and feeling healthy.

Even the most old-school personal trainer has to admit that risk of injury becomes astronomically high when overweight people, who have been sitting all day, start jumping up and loading their untrained body parts in an overhead squat!

Add competitve group dynamics, complex movement patterns, poor diet and lifestyle habits, and a constantly evolving trend of fitness equipment and ideas, and we have millions of little injury power kegs waiting to go off and derail the journey toward fitness.

As a sports physiotherapist servicing a massive local gym for over twenty years, this type of injury was my bread and butter. After a while, my energies inevitably turned to prevention and its importance over some supposed cure. Injuries are here to stay in sports and fitness. But as I asked myself, surely we can reduce the rates of injury frustration in our little neck of the woods through education, screening and intervention to help people stay injury-free?

I believe we can prevent future injury in clients, regardless of whether they currently carry any injury or not. But oils ain't oils, as they say – not everything works. And nothing works as well as the spruikers selling it would like you to think. This is true even for the system we are about to propose, because the real value is found in the quality of coaching – how well you relate to, educate and coach your clients day to day. Our system has a greater power in the hands of intentional and educated personal trainers than physiotherapists or medical professionals, who usually get there too late.

A program for injury screening will be an invaluable tool for you in your coaching, helping you stay aware of injury potential, refining your ability to predict problems and aiding your client's injury prevention.

As the average fitness professional, and the industry as a whole, continues to grow in injury awareness, it will increasingly factor the risks of injury into programs and equipment design. As a functional trainer, it's vital you don't get left behind.

When you got your qualifications in personal training, you probably thought that injuries weren't much of a big deal. Without refining your awareness, you will end up continuing in this mode of thinking, blindly pushing clients toward fitness goals and scratching your frustrated head when problems crop up that could have been prevented. I hope that the research will convince you to take injury awareness on board.

Injury awareness, prediction and prevention are all underpinned by an adequate client screening system. Learning what dysfunctional movement is – and, from that basis, how to screen for it – is the most relevant and practical way to minimise injury in your fitness community. Screening is a systemised way of doing things that keeps you aware, finds those who are at risk, and empowers you to lead your clients to helping themselves reduce their injury risk. If you can screen and predict with some accuracy who will get injured, you can more effectively focus your energies on those clients and their risk factors.

Before looking at how to systematically screen for injury, it's worth clearing up some questions about the sometimes contested issue of injury in fitness. In this chapter, we look at injury statistics, and examine the effectiveness of injury prevention and injury prediction in coaching settings.

Injuries in fitness: what are the statistics?

Chronic pain, overuse and niggling injury – usually leading to frustration from trainer and client – is rampant and hard to quantify due to the vast scale of the fitness industry. It is the dark side of the whole fitness game, which must be faced, not with bravado, but with calm determination.

Make no mistake, individuals with sport or fitness goals regularly get injured. Detailed data on injury incidence specifically in the fitness industry is not in abundance, possibly because injuries are rarely monitored or recorded by operators.[15] However, the limited evidence that is available paints a worrying picture.

Here is some of the research:

> One valuable Australian study closely followed 991 sedentary men and women (aged twenty to sixty-three) for the first four months that they were engaged in a new fitness program. The astounding results were that new injuries were reported by 38% of subjects, with an average duration of impairment of 3.8 weeks, and 43% of those who were injured sought medical treatment. The most frequent types, locations and causes of injury were joint sprains/strains (66%), the lower leg (70%) and jogging (33%).[16]

Take away: 38% of clients engaging in a new fitness program developed injuries within the first four months.

---

15   G Egger, 'Sports injuries in Australia: causes, cost and prevention', *Health Promotion Journal of Australia*, vol. 1, no. 2, 1991, pp. 28–33; BH Jones, DN Cowan and JJ Knapik, 'Exercise, Training and Injuries', *Sports Medicine*, vol. 18, no. 3, 1994, pp. 202–14; Medibank Private 2004, Medibank private sports injuries report, *Medibank Private*, Melbourne.

16   A Sedgwick, D Smith and M Davies, 'Musculoskeletal status of men and women who entered a fitness program', *The Medical Journal of Australia*, vol. 148, no. 8, 1988, pp. 385, 388–91.

About half of the same subjects in the same study reported having received treatment for musculoskeletal ailments previously, or that they were currently experiencing musculoskeletal pain and/or discomfort, and about a third of the subjects reported one or more movement limitations.

Take away: 50% of all people in the study had an injury history of some sort that they had received treatment for.

An investigation into the prior and consequent injury rates of individuals participating in fitness industry programs was carried out with participants of fitness centres and studios in the Bay Area in California. In this study, 70.6% of participants (or 696 of 986) reported one or more previous significant injuries prior to participation in the program, with two or more injury sites reported by 43%, and almost one in ten reporting five or more locations. The rate for all injuries reported during participation was 7.83 per 1,000 hours of activity, or 2.33 injuries per year.[17]

Take away: A whopping 70% of fitness participants had a significant injury history.

A more recent American investigation showed similar outcomes. This study described the types and frequencies of musculoskeletal injuries among a cohort of adults with above-average activity levels who were enrolled in the Aerobics Center Longitudinal Study. A quarter of all participants reported a musculoskeletal injury during the period of participation. Of these, 83% were reported as being activity-related.[18]

Take away: 25% of fit individuals developed an injury during the time of the study!

---

17 RK Requa, LN DeAvilla and JG Garrick, 'Injuries in recreational adult fitness activities', *The American Journal of Sports Medicine*, vol. 21, no. 3, 1993, pp. 461–467.

18 JM Hootman et al., 'Epidemiology of musculoskeletal injuries among sedentary and physically active adults', *Medicine & Science in Sports & Exercise*, vol. 34, no. 5, 2002, pp. 838–44.

Let's think about what these studies tell us.

First, you can pretty much assume that at least a third of people who have been previously sedentary will develop injuries purely from beginning a new training program.

What's more, the same parameters (intensity, duration and frequency) that determine positive fitness and health outcomes from a training program also appear to influence the participant's risk of injuries.

About half of all clients are likely to have some experience with injuries when they begin their fitness program, either carrying them or having had treatment for them at some stage.

Sport participants had the highest proportion of all-cause and activity-related musculoskeletal injuries among both men and women, suggesting that amount and intensity of activity was related to injury development.

From all of this we learn one clear thing. Injuries are a natural side-effect of exercise! That's the reality. So what are we going to do about it?

How effective is injury prevention?

As we have said, our ultimate goal is to help our clients prevent injuries while they strive for fitness goals. Prevention is always better than cure, even if it can be hard to motivate clients (let alone any of us!) to do rehab or corrective exercises before any problem has yet surfaced.

Given these injury rates, prediction and prevention of injury should be one of the highest priorities for clients who are becoming fitness enthusiasts. But many coaches will legitimately ask, 'Is it truly possible to prevent my clients from getting injuries as they increase their training?' We need to look into prevention methods and how effective they actually are.

Injury prevention is in reality an old science, a 'black art' even, that many elite sports professionals claim to have mastered in the name of keeping athletes competing and bringing home the medals. But their athletes do still get injured.

These same professionals will simultaneously acknowledge that it can be very tricky to correlate the injury screening they have performed with strategies that will genuinely prevent injuries occurring during group fitness classes, PT sessions or on the sporting field. We may have screened – but what kind of interventions are best suited to clients?

And then there is the significant matter of whether the intervention actually can be guaranteed to prevent injury anyway.

Despite these questions, the risk of not prescribing injury prevention programs and protocols seems like a risk not worth taking, because – at least anecdotally – prevention programs seem to have higher value, especially where high-value athletes and sporting teams have serious money at stake to keep injury-free, and gyms and personal training businesses have a cumulative financial stake in preventing injury to allow members to keep using their facilities.

Here are a couple of reasons why the science of injury prevention can be such a challenge:

1. TENSION BETWEEN VALUES OF SPORTS PERFORMANCE AND SPORTS MEDICINE

As a fitness professional, you might have experienced this tension yourself: do you *push ahead for fitness and performance*, or *respect an injury and go slow*, knowing how fragile the body is?

One of the main reasons it is difficult to reduce injury risk factors in sports and fitness relates to this tension. There are essential differences in the values of athletes and sporting bodies on the one hand and allied health and medicine on the other. That is, the players and administrators want the stars on the field performing, whereas the medical staff want to minimise the likelihood of re-injury.

This significant tension is clearly experienced on a weekly basis by the coaching staff and players of an AFL team, versus the sports medicine staff. To play or not to play this weekend on that sprained ankle or strained hamstring?

For fitness professionals, and even forward-thinking allied health professionals, the key question is constantly how to progress clients without aggravating an injury: 'Do I allow squatting today with a knee that is in pain getting up and down stairs?' The performance goal of progressing loaded movement is conflicting to some extent with the injury minimisation goals.

To put it another way, if a certain gym member has set aside time for some exercise, will they choose the (often boring) exercises that (hopefully) prevent them getting injured, or will they choose the (fun) exercises that (definitely) help them lose weight or excel in an upcoming competition?

It is an uphill battle, isn't it!

2. THE COMPLEXITY OF THE PROCESS

From start to finish, the process of researching, developing and delivering an effective injury prevention plan for a group or individual is complex. The latest model being used to develop injury prevention strategies is termed the 'TRIPP model' (Translating Research into Injury Prevention Practice). The US Army consistently uses complex protocols like this in its efforts to minimise injury among soldiers.[19]

While it might be challenging to figure out what constitutes effective prevention, there are still a few research studies that back up the value of prescribing exercises for preventing strains and pains for particular groups of active people:

---

19 Read about it yourself by checking out an overview here: http://www.ncbi.nlm.nih.gov/pubmed/10091275, and some of the conclusions: http://www.ncbi.nlm.nih.gov/pubmed/10091275)

- The risk of sustaining an ankle injury among basketball players was reduced by 35.5% (wow!) in an experimental group that performed a series of neuromuscular exercises over the course of a season as part of their weekly training load.[20]

- In a similar study among football players, those who had 'high levels of compliance' had a (massive) 35% lower risk of all injuries compared with players who only had 'intermediate levels of compliance' with the prescribed warm-up program.[21]

- A seven-week off-season program of mobility and stability exercises created a significant improvement in scores for 'Functional Movement Screening' (FMS Gray Cook) for elite footballers. Forty-one players were free of asymmetry post-testing as compared with thirty-one at the pre-test. Note that this could not be extrapolated to say that their injury risk on the football field was any lower. Nevertheless, they were moving with less asymmetry and positive changes took place in movement efficiency.[22]

- In a meta-analysis of recreational sports using warm-up to prevent injury, five high-quality studies were analysed. While the case wasn't strong for the need to warm up, the evidence was still in favour of doing it over not doing it.[23]

Basically, this research all indicates that doing injury prevention is better than *not* doing it. It isn't an exact science, but let's not forget we are screening humans, not machines. Despite the positive research, there

---

20   E Eils, 'Multi-station proprioceptive exercise program prevents ankle injuries in basketball', *Medicine and Science in Sports and Exercise*, vol. 42, no. 11, 2010, pp. 2098–105.

21   T Soligard et al., 'Compliance with a comprehensive warm-up program to prevent injuries in youth football', *British Journal of Sports Medicine*, vol. 44, no. 11, 2010, pp. 787–93.

22   K Kiesel, P Plisky and R Butler, 'Functional movement test scores improve following a standardized off-season intervention program in professional football [gridiron] players', *Scandanavian Journal of Medicine and Science in Sports*, vol. 21, no. 2, 2011, pp. 287–92.

23   AJ Fradkin, BJ Gabbe and PA Cameron, 'Does warming-up prevent injury in sport? The evidence from randomised controlled trials', *Journal of Science and Medicine in Sport*, vol. 9, no. 3, 2006, pp. 214–20.

can never be any guarantee of staying injury-free for this reason: humans are complex.

At the very least, if your client does get injured, you can't say you didn't try to help!

Injury screening and prediction

The final issue to address before launching into a screening protocol is whether it is actually possible to anticipate who will get injured. For this, we need to look at both the forest and the trees.

Broadly speaking, injury screening can be carried out with a whole group or an individual. To be truly accurate and effective, it is advisable to carry out an injury-risk assessment and implement preventative measures at both levels.

Ideally this is done for a group participating in the same sport or fitness activity. Participants are encouraged to be screened at both a 'macro' (group) and a 'micro' (individual) level. Spend all your time on only one of these two and you risk missing critical screening information and delivering poor injury prevention strategies. The macro view takes into acount things like the environment, the group culture and the activity itself, whereas the micro view looks at an individual's biomechanics and injury history.

Generally, sport and fitness cultures are stubborn, funding can be poor and individuals are lazy and tend to focus on the 'fun exercises'. The process of injury screening and prevention takes time and can be boring and complex, and some would argue that for every good study arguing for it, there is one arguing against it. The reality is that very few injury screening and prevention programs have been widely implemented and evaluated to show clear cause-effect relationships. Nonetheless, it is still common practice for sports physiotherapists and biomechanists in developed countries to work with elite teams analysing the musculoskeletal and kinematic status of athletes to look for weaknesses.

It is important to be positive about finding relevant high-risk factors in a client's functional movement and biomechanical system, but also realistic about how good we are (or aren't) at foretelling who will fall apart.

Ultimately, predicting injury and pain is a mysterious space – at some levels we know so little about who will and won't get injured. Watch two middle-aged men training toward a marathon. Or a CrossFit comp. Or a boxing match. Who is to say who will collect an injury and who won't? It is multifactorial beyond belief. Work stresses, previous injury history, dominance, training plan, genetics and many other factors may predispose an individual to injury, and these therefore need to be screened for.

The following table gives a good overview of the different categories that a person or sporting group could be deficient in that would require screening.

Categories Requiring Screening for Sports Injury Prevention[24]

Three Categories of Sport Injury prevention

Training: This includes all forms of physical preparation for sport and exercise
    Muscular strength
    Muscular endurance
    Agility
    Muscular power
    Balance
    Sport-specific skills

Equipment: This includes devices, braces, footwear and surfaces
    Protective equipment
    Foortwear/orthotics
    Gymnasium floors
    Load-bearing surfaces

Regulatory: This includes the rules and regulations that govern sport
    Sport rules
    Association rules
    Legal rules
    Education regarding regulations

---

24   M Klügl et al., 'The prevention of sport injury: an analysis of 12,000 published manuscripts', *Clinical Journal of Sport Medicine*, vol. 20, no. 6, 2010, pp. 407–12.

First, there's the 'forest view'. Many items in this list are simply not relevant for the gym environments where you are working with clients – but why don't you go through with a fine-tooth comb to see which ones are? Is your physical environment relevant? Is the culture created in some group exercise classes negative toward injuries being mentioned? Which equipment isn't conducive to good form? This is subject to interpretation (and even an element of mystery), yet it's worthwhile figuring out which components of your chosen program, equipment and culture could be most relevant for minimising injury.

Then there's the 'tree view'. The most complex element that requires screening is the actual functioning of a client's body movements. Our system for helping you spot high-risk ingredients in how clients move, which we delve into in the following chapter, is both common sense (for example, clearly highlighting areas of pain) and also biomechanically complex (for example, figuring out how to decide if your client's thoracic spine is too stiff for overhead press).

When it comes to anticipating injury, the biggest take away is that clients with no injury history are easier to predict. Many agree that *the biggest predictor of future injury is past injury history*, with the understanding that small remnants of the old injury will always hang around, ready to stage a potential comeback. So, if a client reports no niggling or serious pain, or even much of a history of injury, then screening them and predicting if they are going to get injured (and preventing them from becoming injured) seems a little easier to forecast.

Are you injury aware?

Overall, you could say that the *anecdotal* evidence for injury screening and prevention (historical experience, generally accepted wisdoms, common practice) is stronger than the statistical research. But isn't that the story for most of what we call effective corrective exercise, allied health and medicine? No research will beat years of experience and intuitive, honest engagement with human bodies struggling to improve their functional and sporting performance.

Even if there is no guarantee that we can pick up through screening every client who will get injured, let's not give up trying! Clients love the extra levels of care and intentionality given to them, and it keeps us aware of all the subtle risks of injury that are the natural side-effects of pushing the body hard into new realms of fitness.

Injury prevention strategies such as improved warm-ups and self-care corrective exercises are no rock-solid guarantee either, but they are much better than blindly rushing ahead.

We just want to get those statistics down from one third to no thirds, don't we? Fewer and fewer clients getting injured when they start their fitness programs with us – that's what we are striving hard toward. Over the next two chapters, we will look at injury prevention strategies and how to implement them.

After all, prevention is better than cure.

Effective Injury Screening

What is dysfunctional movement?

At one level, all movement is 'functional'. Humans must move to live and thrive, rather than be sedentary. Therefore, excessive sitting and lack of activity is the essence of 'dysfunctional movement' for the human body.

But it's also true that much human movement is not ideal, and that even where certain forms of movement allow a person to perform a function, these patterns themselves can still be dysfunctional. Compensatory patterns are dysfunctional: they are effectively a 'second-rate option for movement' that the brain learns to normalise.

There are many complex dysfunctional movements that occur during vigorous exercise, and this requires us to drill down into how an individual moves: how their particular body lifts something from the floor, loads onto one leg, carries something heavy or stands for a long period of time. To be brutally honest, most human movement is at least a bit dysfunctional! Compensatory movement is actually normal, but that shouldn't stop us screening for it to prevent and minimise injury.

Dysfunctional movement refers to elements along the human kinetic chain (joints, muscles and fascia that are anatomically linked together) being overloaded or underloaded. Muscles are understood to be ineffective to do the tasks they are designed to do. The common, well-documented pattern is that:

- Firstly, stabilising muscles that have a more supportive role and use lower contraction thresholds for longer periods of time seem to regress and underwork, becoming inhibited and dormant.

- Concurrently, power muscles that rapidly contract to create movement are potentially hypertonic (highly activated) and overwork. They may assume the role of false stabiliser over time if the postural muscles do not get retrained effectively.

- Lastly, joints, fascia and nerve tissue are overloaded in directions that destroy their integrity and bring on early breakdown.

This overloading and underloading of multiple tissues along the kinetic chain leads to gradual build up of pain and injury.

There's no doubt that every client has some level of dysfunctional joint, muscle and fascial movement, negatively affecting their functional training. Your clients are doing functional training dysfunctionally somehow or other, and you need to screen them to bring that to the light and into the conversation.

We have all watched as new types of functional equipment and techniques have begun transforming the world of fitness over the last quarter of a century. Exercise prescriptions are increasingly 'functional' in that they are meaningful to clients' needs, and the equipment and training programs are better at working with the body's primal movement patterns – the basic, natural patterns of human movement. On a global scale, there is no doubt that the fitness industry has evolved to improve movement quality over this time.

However, despite this trend, dysfunctional movement continues unabated among certain groups, fitness cultures and individuals, and addressing it requires you as a coach to have a focus on function. Instead of focusing purely on the end goal of a movement pattern, you need to ask a different question.

Forget asking, 'What's your personal best for a 5 km run?' Ask instead, 'How is your running – how efficient, how smooth, how easy?' Ask, 'How did the run feel?' And instead of asking, 'Can you squat 150 kgs?' ask, 'Was your back sore for the next two to three days?' – a question more concerned about load distribution, joint control and lumbar spine safety than numbers. Same goes for push-ups, overhead presses, lunges and any exercise you can think of.

At this point, some of the sharper folk among you may want to counter these ideas with some very good questions, so let me see if I can effectively answer them!

Q: Are compensatory movements ever viewed positively? If someone is born with a clear deviation or discrepancy, whether large (like a missing limb) or barely discernable (like a hip retroversion that causes hip and foot to flare out), and they've lived their whole life adapted to this pattern without pain, is it positive or negative?

A: The reality is that some compensatory movements are more destructive than others, and the longer the body has had time to adapt, the less impact they will have. So genetic elements such as the retroverted hip will be well adapted to, and problems may only arise later on through life events such as injuries or sports. If someone has no pain, this may not be due to them adapting well so much as their healthy psychology or physiology, which also impacts on injury rates.

Q: Are there times when adaptations should just be left alone rather than corrected? Could trying to 'correct' in the above situation, for example, lead to injury?

A: I think all dysfunctional movements are open to correction, unless you are dealing with an 'elite' athlete and two things exist: minimal pain levels and critically high levels of demand during a season. So, in that example you would only ever seek to correct a movement problem with a motivated athlete during off-season.

Q: How can a trainer discern what is a maladaptation and what is a healthy and workable compensation?

A: I think at this point it is safest to consider all compensations as maladaptive. There is no doubt, however, than in correcting many dysfunctional patterns you will come up against a deeper blockage in the movement. For example, in trying to minimise posterior tilt at the pelvis, the hip joint may be discovered to be very tight and even painful at certain angles.

Your job is to coach your client to awareness and knowledge of their injury (potential or actual) and toward responsibility and commitment in managing and overcoming it. In this chapter we'll look at the three layers of dysfunctional movement to get a deeper understanding of what could be going on for your client. Then we'll look at the three-part dysfunctional movement screen we use as part of the Adaptive FTS.

The three layers of dysfunction

How can you know in a concrete way if and how your client is moving dysfunctionally? How should you assess, record and manage compensatory movements for your clients? When setting clients up for functional movement training, what factors do you look for to reduce the injury risk enough to justify the effort? Unless all of these questions are addressed through adequate screening and coaching, your training regimen may promote new injury or aggravation of existing or old injuries.

We look for three possible layers (or types) of dysfunction that prevent healthy functional movement and create compensatory movements, regardless of the training program or equipment used:

- The presence of pain
- Biomechanical blockages
- Bad habits of movement

Which element is the chicken and which is the egg? For example, is the client medially deviating at the knee due to a biomechanical blockage at the hip, or is pain in the knee inhibiting muscle stability and causing medial knee deviation and eventual biomechanical changes in the hip? Or is one of the three – let's say the knee pain is due to a cut or bump – happening in isolation?

There are multiple possible relationships between these three powerful destroyers of functional movement, but without doubt the presence of pain is the most intense for the human body.

Surprisingly, some people have extremely obvious bad habits of movement or biomechanical blockages, but never get pain, while others seem to get pain at the drop of a hat without either of the other two being present.

Mostly though, the three elements feed into each other and take up a dance of sorts. Pain may lead to (or be caused by) biomechanical blockages; bad movement habits may predispose to pain and/or biomechanical blockages. They are linked to different degrees in different people.

PRESENCE OF PAIN

Regardless of which comes first, pain (and the fear of it) is the most powerful 'wrecking ball' of functional movement. It creates a cascade of negative effects, including bad movement habits and eventual biomechanical blockage.It is a lot like sticking a screwdriver into the cogs of a well-oiled machine and watching it come to a grinding halt. Whether the pain is deep or superficial, vague or sharp, intense or mild, it will negatively affect the client's movement and make it dysfunctional.

While a full explanation of the neurochemical complexity of pain is beyond the scope of this book, the key thing to grasp is that pain causes a powerful protective reaction that forces movement away from that painful region or joint area. Early in the brain's process of self-protection, certain stability or postural muscles are quick to become 'inhibited' subconsciously, exacerbating the feeling of weakness of the area to the conscious mind. The brain then begins directing movement traffic away from the painful region to allow the whole body to continue to move around the area that is recovering.

Most body regions have multiple second-rate options (compensations) for movement, which are designed to deload the painful area for the short term but are less than optimal as a strategy for the medium to long term. Such compensations are not the ideal way to move; they are neither efficient, nor are they classically functional. Most of them sit under the umbrella term 'bad habits of movement', which we look at later. Here are some examples:

- **Scenario 1:** An injury to a client's knee causes the brain to shunt more load through the low back during any bending movements. In this situation, hip and lumbar flexion become the preferred movement to protect the knee. This works fine for a short period of time to protect the knee, but it is not long before the low back feels the strain and may begin to break down in soft tissue overload or in neuromuscular function.

- **Scenario 2:** A client receives a small whiplash from being rear-ended while driving, resulting in neck pain. This will commonly result in excessive elevation of the shoulder in order to take load off the neck and allow it to heal. After a while, however, it may result in overactivity in those muscles (upper trapezius, levator scapulae, and rhomboids) resulting potentially in longer-term changes in the brain and what is commonly termed 'muscle imbalance'.

- **Scenario 3:** A client with a sore shoulder struggles to hold form while preforming overhead presses. Discomfort in the shoulder near the top of the movement will cause the brain to avoid this part of the movement, instead shearing the pelvis and lumbar spine forward and creating stress and overload to fragile joint structures in that region.

Interestingly, it is unlikely to be the actual pain that is the issue in many more-chronic situations, but rather the fear of it. Extensive research on the link of fear to chronic low back pain by medical researchers has shed light on this reality.[25] It is the fear that locks the brain into longer-term bad habits of movement, even long after the painful area has healed.

---

25   M Grotle et al., 'Fear-avoidance beliefs and distress in relation to disability in acute and chronic low back pain', *Pain*, vol. 112 no. 3, 2004, pp. 343–52.

Shopping in a local hardware shop a while back, I was asked by the attendant if I would be able to pick up the materials on the ground floor by bringing my car to the lower entrance. 'As long as you feel confident to reverse down a long narrow alleyway,' he remarked. 'Sure!' I said, and the job was done. Reversing a car is something I am very confident in doing, so it was no problem – but it struck me how important it was that I had confidence in the movement in order to execute it well, and the attendant and I chatted about that for five minutes. Hmmm, I thought.

An hour later, I was working with my father to paint the roof of my house, and I hate heights – I'm so afraid of falling. I was astounded at the lack of confidence in my movements compared to my dad, seventy-six years old and moving like a cat across a sloping roof, ten metres above the ground! Just knowing we were that high up, I simply couldn't move properly. The fear froze my brain and muscles, placing me at serious risk of falling. My lack of confidence wrecked my movement completely.

This incident brought to my attention how our fears destroy our confidence. The same goes for our clients when we are training them. What might we or our clients be afraid of that negatively influences our functional movement?

Fear of pain is the greatest obstacle for clients of personal trainers. It is the biggest threat, hands down, to your clients staying on the fitness journey with you. Take stock of how you talk to your clients, how you motivate them and how you push them. Never use fear as your tool, because it takes away your clients' confidence in themselves and how well they are doing. Poor movement will be the result.

Movement without fear is a key to regaining confidence and a necessary part of rehabilitation of an injury. Are there ways you can encourage clients to 'rehearse the movement without pain'?

BIOMECHANICAL BLOCKAGES

Where there is injury to fragile joint, tendon, capsular or nerve structures, the brain's response is to 'lock down' those areas, rendering them relatively immobile while the tissues heal. This immobility that allows healing may last from a few days to many months, depending on the extent of the damage and also whether surgery has been required.

The longer the time off from healthy movement, the longer the time and energy required to restore it. A joint or region will often regain some of its mobility and neuromuscular coordination quite naturally as life returns to normal, but whether it will regain enough of it for functional movement to be restored is another matter altogether. Most commonly, residual joint hypomobility (stiffness), fascial and neural hypersensitivity (pain) and muscular imbalance will remain.

These underlying negative changes, which soon feel normal, are often disguised behind a new compensatory pattern as pain ceases. The biomechanical blockage has gone into hiding beneath new bad movement habits, becoming increasingly locked into the human biomechanical system. Here it sits below the surface like an iceberg that threatens to sink a ship, only coming into view as movement gets underway with exercise.

Hidden biomechanical blockages within movement patterns are resistant to change due to the complex web of joint, muscular, fascial and neural (both local to the area and in the brain) changes that have set in. They are critical to bring to the client's attention, yet this can be tricky due to the nature of the problem – they have often been brilliantly compensated for. Clients must see clearly how one side of their body, or one particular movement, is simply blocked. It may bring up pain to push load into or simply be too stiff to push through, but often it's tricky to pinpoint due to its hidden nature.

Here are three examples of what biomechanical blockages might look like:

Scenario 1: A small ankle sprain that prevented a client from running for a month has resulted in a stiffness. Ever so subtly, the client now loads differently through the leg (a new bad movement habit). What is left is a blockage of 10–20% to normal dorsiflexion of the ankle (the forward movement of the knee beyond the toes when weight bearing) with consequent increase in hip flexion during their squat and lunging exercises and an increase in load through their lumbar spine.

Scenario 2: A season of heavy training for a tennis competition has resulted in a new tightness in a client's right shoulder (without pain). Consequently, they are now unable to get as vertical with their arm during a kettlebell overhead press. Wrist pain and neck pain on that side are creeping in after their kettlebell sessions. Again, a new bad movement habit has crept in to compensate for the biomechanical blockage (see same example later).

Scenario 3: Longer hours at the computer have stiffened a client's thoracic spine such that full extension is now reduced. The client's head is now sitting slightly forward of their collarbones and increased load is felt through the neck, with occasional headaches resulting.

BAD HABITS OF MOVEMENT

Humans move with habituated patterns that become normalised through repetition. Those of us with minimum disruption in our human development will move quite functionally, with few obvious bad habits. However, most of us are affected early on in our development or later in life by factors that set us up for dysfunctional movement. These include:

Genetics – Very few of us are not born with some genetic (also termed 'structural') deviance from the average. We may be born with a slight scoliosis, increased scapular winging, knee valgus (medial position) or a flat back. We adapt to these unique elements, and they in themselves rarely give us any trouble unless our environment changes through injury or new lifestyle ingredients.

Left/right dominance – A normal preference for arm or leg use may become prominent by habituation or through injury where the body needs to protect an injured side. When normal mild asymmetry becomes more pronounced, overload can be the result. This overload will exacerbate any mild bad movement habits that are present through genetics, sports or work.

Sports – Long seasons of any sports will slowly create bad habits of movement even while we are becoming more skilled, fit or flexible. This is due to the nature of focusing so heavily on one activity. Hockey will cause increased anterior tilt at the pelvis with all the forward bending; netball easily allows for medial knee jarring; tennis leads to poor push/pull movements such as winging of the scapula, and so on. Even complex, high-level sports like gymnastic sees young athletes riddled with subtle bad movement habits that lead many to quit early due to multiple niggling injuries.

Work – Increased demands on the body at work will strengthen and tighten arms, legs or trunk in certain imbalanced ways, just as sports do.

Injuries – Injuries are by far the most powerful dictator of movement changes. The brain shuts down certain movements that cause pain and works around them through compensation. The brain then slowly becomes used to such patterns, which are normalised through repetition. Any other factors will be sidelined immediately as there is no more powerful destroyer of movement patterns than pain.

Client's body awareness – Not all clients are created equal in terms of their ability to feel, perceive and understand their own movement, and therefore some may drift into bad habits without any recognition.

They may be very tight in certain areas or genetically hypermobile. In either case they may be without pain, but due to unawareness be very prone to, and difficult to train out of, bad movement habits.

Training errors – While this opinion is somewhat controversial, we believe that certain exercises, if taught excessively or in isolation, will actually cause dysfunctional movement. These faulty movement choices, often taught to clients as 'functional', can easily result in overtraining, as they require the body to unlearn natural movements or learn unnatural movements. Examples of these include:

- Bench press (restricts scapular movement and overloads the rotator cuff)

- Overhead squat (forces the client to learn the unnatural element of pushing overhead while descending into the deep squat – multiple problems may result)

- Push/pull movements with no scapular movement (keep shoulders back and down the whole time)

- Squats where knees are kept behind the line of the toes (poor quadricep activation, poor dorsiflexion, lumbar spine overload result)

- Full range deep squats where the client is unable to perform these easily in a bodyweight movement

- Overhead press where arm is kept in internal rotation at the top of the movement (increased shoulder impingement risk)

- Loading with excessive fatigue and insufficient recovery (clients struggle to move well due to tightness or DOMS)

- Poor equipment choices such as poor shoe selection or excessive wear on shoes

Scenario 1: The small ankle sprain we discussed earlier causes the brain to avoid pure ankle dorsiflexion, which over time becomes the new normal during closed kinetic chain movement. Instead there may be increased anterior or posterior tilt at the pelvis, a Trendelenburg sign and medial knee movement to compensate (which we'll look at further in a moment). In quite a few training environments, clients are taught not to take their knees beyond the line of the toes, which would support the client's inability to do so due to poor dorsiflexion and lead to imbalanced movement patterns.

Scenario 2: The tennis player with shoulder impingement learns to overextend in his wrist and protract his chin further. He may increasingly demonstrate poor pull and push movement as his shoulder is gradually unable to do full and strong scapular retraction and protraction. Use of the bar in back squats will contribute to normalising this, as the restrictions in scapular movement will require increased wrist extension and chin protraction.

Scenario 3: The computer geek with stiff thoracic spine will normalise poor pull movement as she is positioned in increased kyphosis, and will protract her chin and demonstrate increased lordosis in the lumbar spine during overhead movements. Excessive training of abdominal curls or poor warm-up of a thoracic spine that is stiff from the workday will exacerbate this.

As you can see, the root cause of dysfunctional movement is complex. Maladapted movements arise due to the presence of pain, biomechanical blockages or bad movement habits. Any of these individually, or most likely a combination, will constitute dysfunctional movement and set the client up for future injury.

The injury prevention screen

A thorough screening system is required in order to highlight where the client's movement is being compromised. Our injury prevention screen is made up of three components: TALK, SEE and DO.[26] These components reflect the earlier three layers of dysfunctional movement.

We describe our screening protocol as somewhat similar to the way you are screened at an airport before you can get on a flight. The key question you are trying to solve is this: *Is your client safe to fly?*

ONLINE RESOURCE: Download the IPK recording form from our resource link – http://functionaltraininginstitute.com/book-resources/

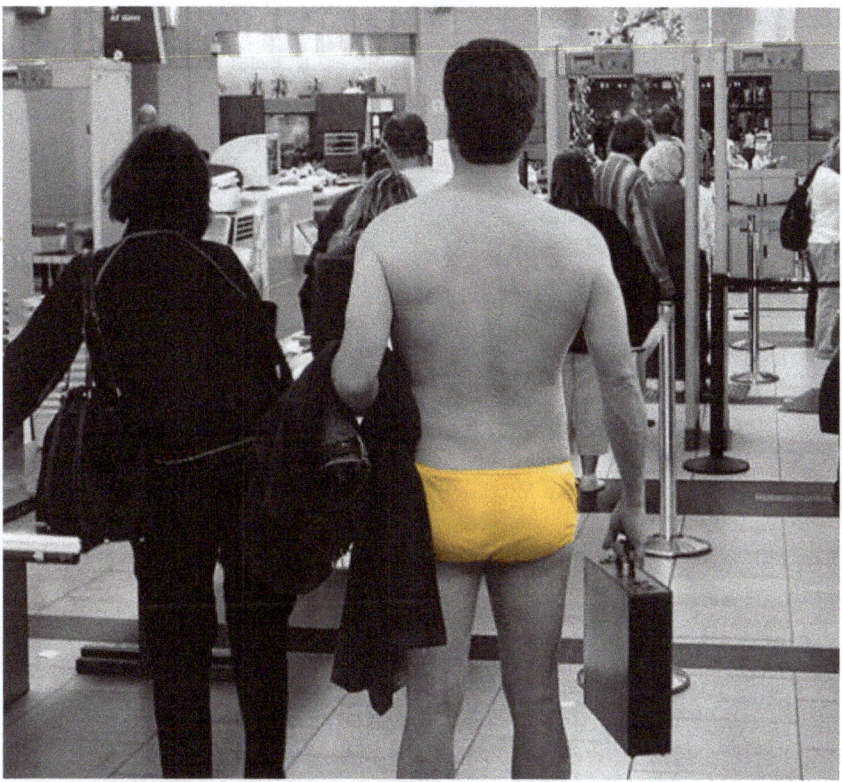

26 Our injury prevention screen is part of the Injury Prevention Kit (IPK) that we teach in the Movement Restoration Coach certification, created and endorsed by Rehab Trainer. More information about this can be found at www.functionaltraininginstitute.com/movement-restoration-coach/

The three airport screening elements a passenger faces are questioning, an X-ray and a bag search.

- **Questioning:** When booking a ticket, you are questioned about whether you are carrying forbidden, inflammable or dangerous goods. You will receive a more serious interview in a separate room later if unidentified substances are detected. This is equivalent to the interview for presence of pain (**TALK**).

- **X-ray:** Passing through the X-ray machine means taking a look at things from an external and objective perspective. This is akin to observation of bad habits of movement (**SEE**).

- **Bag search:** If needed, an in-depth bag search is performed to uncover anything that looked a little strange on the X-ray. This is the equivalent to the ScreenTraining for biomechanical blockages (**DO**).

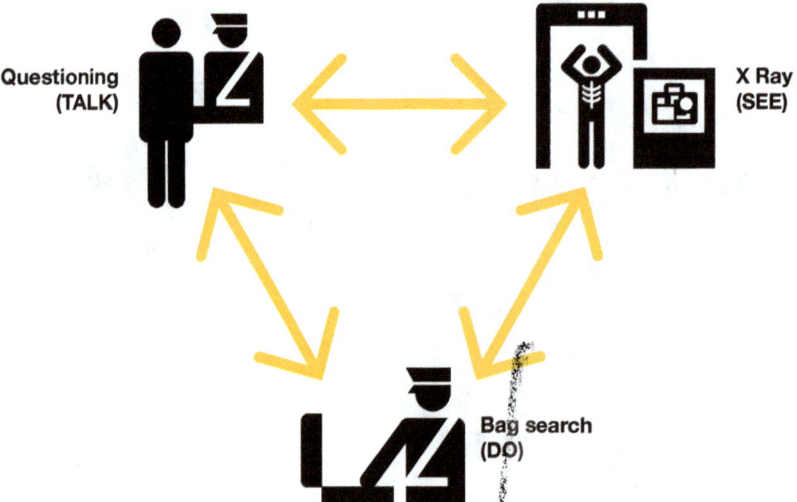

TALK, SEE, DO: these three screening tactics exist like a whirlpool that you enter with the client. Any of the three elements may be a priority, depending on the unique journey of the client, and you enter the screening from that point.

- If the client is keen to TALK about their injuries begin with effective interviewing, then move to either of the other two tactics.

- If the client isn't in pain but moves poorly, then enter through the SEE skill and carefully observe their movement.

- And if the client needs to be assessed for hidden biomechanical blockages then use DO by taking your client through the appropriate ScreenTraining skill (which we're about to go through).

You are likely already doing some of these things. It is quite intuitive for most trainers to watch clients move, chat to them about problems and do some formal assessment. But now there is a clear system that allows room for educating your clients, holding them accountable, inspiring them and generally keeping their commitment to the process sufficient to reduce risk and prevent further injury.

Now let's unpack the three screening tactics further.

TALK: EFFECTIVE INTERVIEWING FOR THE PRESENCE OF PAIN

Multiple chit-chats happen around injuries within the fitness/personal training world, but they are often vague and not constructive to client or trainer confidence in any real way. These chats about injuries see some clients always complaining about or discussing their injuries, and others determined to keep information to themselves to avoid having their injuries take centre stage and wreck their confidence.

Effective interviewing ensures clients are guided through telling their injury story in a way that gives you enough useful information and lets them feel that you care enough to ask real questions.

Confidence is the key to interviewing clients: both your confidence as a coach that things are part of a process that has a meaningful goal, and your client's confidence that the tough patch will pass, and they will eventually be restored to their best function given enough steady effort and time. Maintaining and growing confidence is, hands down, the greatest challenge through injury.

First, ensure you have a quiet space to allow you to concentrate on both the client and their injury, allowing at least five to fifteen minutes for the discussion to take place.

At FTI, we train coaches to become adept in two styles of interview.[27]

First, there is the **Quick TALK**. The goals of interviewing here are to learn three key elements about your client's injury:

1. **Where is the pain?** Where and what exactly are they feeling? Get clients to show with their hands on their body where the pain is while you complete the Body Chart on the IPK Recording Form. Draw in the areas of pain, with descriptions such as 'deep', 'sharp', 'achey', 'tightness'. Check if they experience any pins and needles or numbness.

2. **History of the pain?** Ask for a brief history of their problem or injury, including how long ago and how exactly it happened.

3. **Behaviour of the pain?** Ask how the injury is behaving. What makes symptoms better? What makes them worse?

Then there is the **In-Depth_TALK**. At FTI, we use a more thorough multiple-page questionnaire that seeks to get the full picture of the client's current and past injury history, sport, work and medical factors, and future goals.

From either the Short TALK or the In-Depth TALK, a subjective rating of pain intensity is requested on a 0–10 scale of pain experience:

---

[27] For those who undertake our Movement Restoration Coach certification, we provide printable client questionnaires as part of the Injury Prevention Kit (IPK).

- 0 = nothing
- 10 = worst you can imagine!
- For 1–5, rate client as +
- For 6–10, rate client as ++

SEE: DEEP OBSERVATION OF BAD MOVEMENT HABITS

All personal trainers watch their clients move, but most do not know what they are looking for – what dysfunctional movements look like to the observing eye. Deep observance of how a client moves forms the basis of screening for bad movement habits. It is a skill that takes practice, especially for subtle variations in the athlete who has learned to move well despite such habits (although the clock is always ticking in these situations).

Look especially for subtle difference between right and left sides. This asymmetry reveals old protective or compensatory patterns that must be brought to light, graded (as mild + or obvious ++), explained to the client, mirrored back if needed, video recorded and generally brought to attention as an issue. Offering feedback to the client in training sessions and regularly taking them aside to screen again is all part of coaching them in their efforts to unlearn these patterns.

There are seven bad movement habits that we consider critical to notice, each best understood in the context of a certain type of exercise or technique drill such as a squat or pull movement.[28]

They are:

1. Medial knee deviation in the lunge or squat
2. The Trendelenburg sign in gait, running, or single-leg standing positions
3. Hyper-lordosis in straight-body positions

---

28 We cover these movements extensively, with supporting video materials, in our Movement Restoration Coach certification.

4. Excessive posterior tilt in the squat or deadlift
5. A 'lurching' or winged scapula in the push movement
6. A 'lurching' or lifting scapula in the pull movement
7. A protracted chin in any loaded position

We are not going to cover all these bad movement habits in detail here, but let me give you a few examples of what they look like:

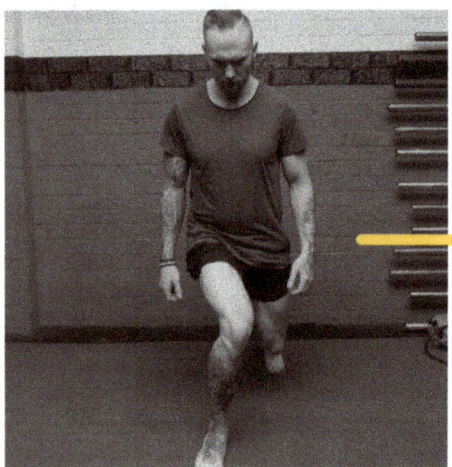 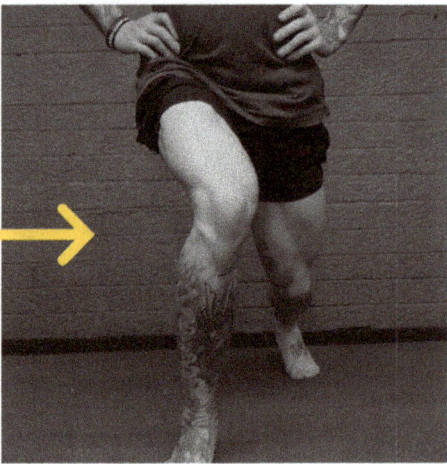

[Seeing an obvious (++) medial knee deviation during the lunge]

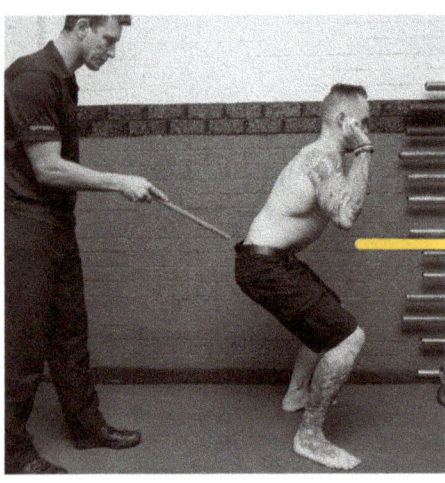 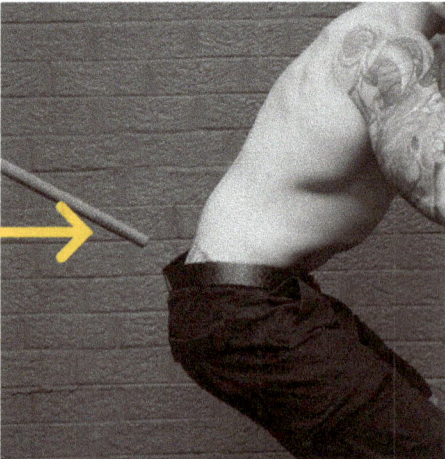

[Seeing a more subtle (+) excessive posterior tilt in squat]

At FTI, we record the client's bad habit of movement and assess it as mild (+) or very obvious (++) on the IPK Recording Form:

DO: SCREENTRAINING FOR BIOMECHANICAL BLOCKAGES

The third component of our injury prevention screen, DO, contains seven very precise movements that are used to screen for a combination of joint stiffness, myofascial restriction, motor control deficiencies, inhibited movements and weakness. We calls these 'ScreenTrains'. They are designed to bring to the surface the hidden icebergs that block good biomechanics, and are therefore done poorly by clients who need to compensate around those blockages. One biomechanical element, or many, may be assessed in one particular ScreenTrain, and are given a + if there is no pain and a ++ if there is pain with the movement.

The seven ScreenTrains are:

1. Supinated ankle
2. Sumo hold
3. Flamingo
4. Hop to quad stretch
5. Waiters bow/butt wink
6. Thoracic killer
7. Airport controller

For example, ScreenTrain #3, the flamingo, challenges hip mobility (posterior hip – the piriformis muscle and hip capsule) concurrently with hip stability on the balancing leg. Not easy!

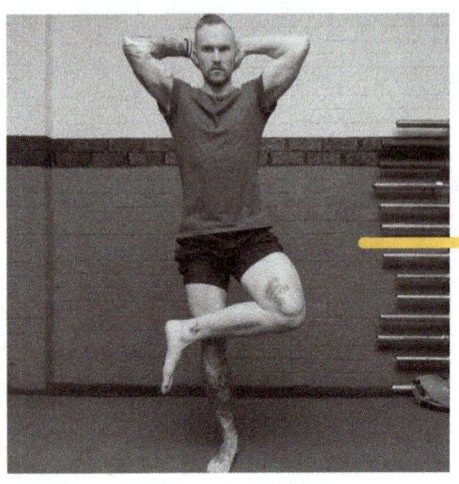
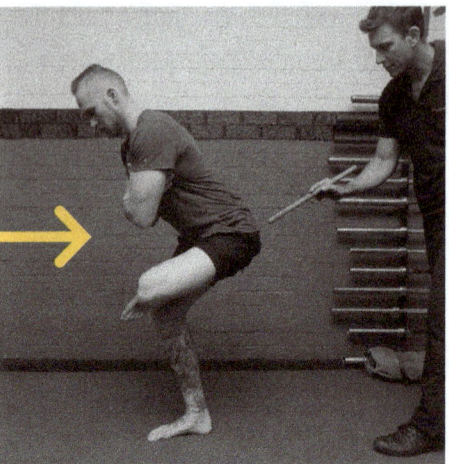

And ScreenTrain #6, affectionately termed the 'thoracic killer', assesses one's ability to extend the upper thoracic spine. (However, it is easy to perform this incorrectly by lifting the chin away from throat – there is always a cheat movement to be aware of!)

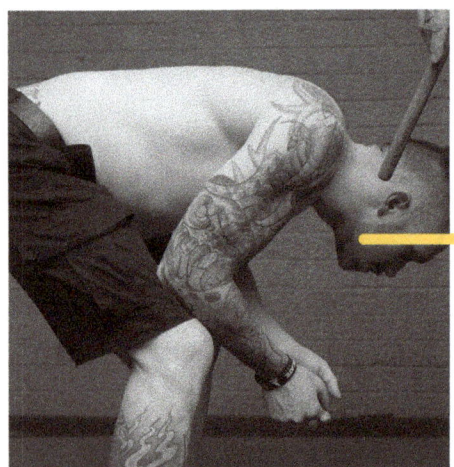
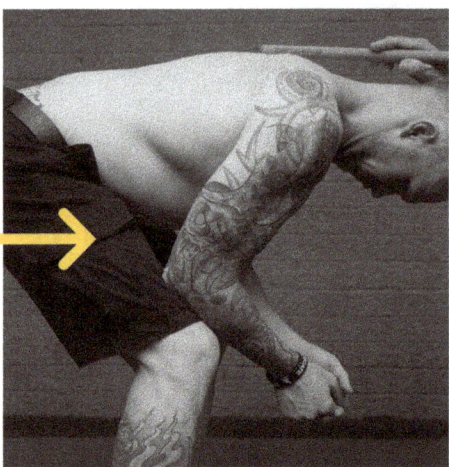

ScreenTrain, no pain? If your client does not experience pain during screening, the screen movement may then become the training movement – hence the term 'ScreenTrain'. The test becomes the training drill. The client is then encouraged to practise the ScreenTrain multiple times per day, their body learning the skill, gaining the mobility and growing in the control required to eventually complete it to your satisfaction.

ScreenTrain, pain? When a client is in pain or unable to complete the ScreenTrain, this will begin the journey toward cleaning up that movement using any modalities (physiotherapy, chiropractic, osteopathy, deep tissue massage, stretching, self myofascial release) that they may choose or that you recommend. Eventually the pain should recede and the ScreenTrain should become easier to practise until it is completed satisfactorily.

Be a champion of injury prevention

Clients, regardless of their state of injury, benefit tremendously from coaches who intentionally play a part in their injury prevention team. Clients who experience an injury-aware trainer become, and stay, motivated to improve their movement and function, even if they are currently seeing health care professionals for an injury and unable to do certain exercises.

Be sure to incorporate 'injury prevention' into your coaching philosophy, values and vision, letting it infiltrate your culture and the way you connect with and challenge clients. Here are some examples of how to do this in a holistic way:

- **Culture:** Make healthy movement and injury prevention part of your value set. This will have a flow-on effect within the whole gym community, where those who are working on their dysfunctional movements are esteemed and given positive feedback and even rewards. When injury prevention becomes part of the language and clients see that poor movement is not denied or shamed, but postively engaged with and corrected, you have changed your culture.

- **Purpose:** Make injury prevention a clear aim for your client. Educate, educate, educate – teach your client about bad movement patterns and how to fix them until the ideas are completely ingrained. If they are posterior-tilting too much, ensure they know exactly how to do the 'waiter's bow' ScreenTrain and are *not* doing it during deadlifting, kettlebell swings or even during squatting in the early stages. Document their purpose somewhere. Review videos taken, write it up on whiteboards.

- **Community relatedness:** Join your client with others working on similar goals. You could even help them form small private Facebook groups for people with similar movement dysfunctions. Get them messaging each other and holding each other to account. Create a fun atmosphere to help feelings of belonging because they are working on a 'weakness' with others.

- **Modelling:** If you are not becoming more functional in your own movement, how can you expect a client to do it? Model how you manage your own body by ensuring that you apply the knowledge and skills to yourself! Feel, see and address your own dysfunctional movements, whether they are due to aches and pains, bad habits or biomechanical blockages. Show clients you are diligently working on your own body.

The journey from dysfunctional movement (especially if pain is present) is quite slow and can easily lead to client discouragement and drop-out. As a coach who champions injury awareness and prevention, you will be positioned perfectly to prevent this from happening, instead keeping clients motivated, educated, inspired and on track for getting the results they seek.

Part 3: Move with Purpose

The 5 Pillars of Functional Training

Pillar 1 – Restore Function and Movement

Restoring function and movement is the advisable first step for anyone embarking on a training program. It is therefore the first pillar in the Adaptive FTS.

Awareness is key. As we explored in Part 1: Coach with Purpose, your coaching skills are sharpened when you empower your clients to be present and mindful, therefore increasing their bodily awareness. At the same time, you increase your own awareness by focusing on the progress of the client.

This pillar draws on your coaching skills of presence and awareness and your capacity to accurately assess movement in order to incorporate restoration and improved movement into a client's program, according to need.

As we have discovered in Part 2: Assess with Purpose, clients will invariably come to you with niggly injuries ('I woke up with a pinch in my shoulder'), poor exercise regimens and chronically bad posture due to lifestyle habits and workplace environments. These common challenges are not the only reason for poor movement; we must take into account past injuries and pathologies that may result in movement dysfunction as well as deeper issues that are not the realm of fitness and health coaches.

The number one goal for coaches is to get clients to optimal movement. Emphasis needs to be placed on progressing clients from dysfunction to optimal movement. Where are they along this continuum?

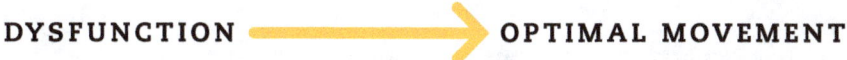

DYSFUNCTION ⟶ **OPTIMAL MOVEMENT**

The movements we will explore here in Pillar 1 form part of the ongoing client screening, which we looked at in Part 2, *Assess with Purpose*. In the Adaptive FTS, we place great emphasis on the need for *ongoing* assessment and screening. Before getting into the components of our mobility sequence, it's worth exploring some questions about mobility.

Common questions

Over our years of teaching mobility to trainers and coaches, there are several questions that pop up with great regularity. While not claiming to cover every curiosity about mobility, the following Q&A is a useful summary and guide to understanding the relevance mobility plays in coaching clients.

What muscles does mobility work target?

We can categorise muscles as 'global' or 'local'. These categories are based on the muscle's functional ability.

Local muscles are thought to be important in joint stability by acting close to the joint axis, providing more joint compression than torque. Local muscles have the ability to stiffen the joint by their large attachments to key passive elements of the joint.[29] The major local muscles include the:

- Deep cervical flexors
- Rotator cuff
- Rhomboids
- Mid and lower trapezius
- Transversus abdominis
- Multifidus
- Diaphragm
- Muscles of the pelvic floor

---

29 Timothy Retchford, 'Can local muscles augment stability in the hip? A narrative literature review', *Journal of musculoskeletal and neuronal interactions*, vol. 13, 2013, pp.1–12.

- Gluteus medius and minimus
- External rotators of the hip
- Vastus medialis obliquus

In contrast, global muscles are more superficial muscles that can generate greater force at joints as a result of their larger physiological cross-sectional area.[30] The major global muscles include the:

- Sternocleidomastoid
- Upper trapezius
- Levator scapulae
- Pectoralis major
- Deltoid
- Latissimus dorsi
- Rectus abdominis
- External obliques
- Erector spinae
- Gluteus maximus
- Hamstrings
- Rectus femoris
- Iliopsoas
- Adductors
- Gastrocnemius/soleus

Local muscles usually require strengthening when it comes to corrective exercises, while global muscles are more likely to be tight and overactive and usually require stretching.[31]

What is the difference between mobility and flexibility?

Mobility is smooth movement: controlled, balanced movement without physical interference. It can be affected by inefficient motor unit coordination or recruitment (neuromuscular), muscle weakness, strength

---

30 Ibid

31 P Page, C Frank and R Lardner, Assessment and treatment of muscle imbalance: the Janda approach, Champaign IL, Human Kinetics, 2010.

asymmetry or joint instability (strength), and joint immobility or muscle tightness. Where mobility targets joints and the flow of movement, flexibility looks at the range of motion available at a joint or group of joints and is often limited by muscle length or tension.

What is stability?

Stability is the neuromuscular system's ability to hold still a part of the body (whether proximal or distal) or to control a stable base during movement. Joint stability maintains a proper alignment of the bony partners of any joint using passive and dynamic components.[32]

Should I stretch? If so, when?

The different types of stretching include static, dynamic and pre-contraction (PNF) methods; all of these types of stretching are equally effective at improving flexibility and muscle extensibility.[33]

Dynamic stretching is the most beneficial type to use before strength and explosive-based exercise. Static stretching may assist with muscle recovery and therefore is most beneficial after exercise; it is not ideal before speed, power and strength training, as it 'relaxes' muscles and can lead to reduced performance.

What causes DOMS and what is the best way to reduce it?

Contrary to common opinions, lactic acid does not cause delayed-onset muscle soreness (DOMS). It's usually caused by unaccustomed exercise, particularly exercise that requires primarily eccentric muscle action. The eccentric action occurs when a muscle generates tension to control the rate it lengthens. Typically, the soreness arises within the first day after exercise and peaks in intensity at around forty-eight hours. According

---

[32] C Kisner and LA Colby, Therapeutic exercise: foundations and techniques, Philadelphia, FA Davis, 2012.
[33] Page et al, Ibid.

to current research, there is no strong evidence that muscle stretching reduces DOMS in any clinically important way in healthy adults. The most efficient methods to prevent or reduce DOMS include:

- Gradual exposure to eccentric-based exercise through incrementally increasing the intensity of a new exercise program (known as 'the repeated bout effect')[34]
- Wearing of compression garments during and immediately after exercise and up to three days following[35]
- Self-myofascial release via the use of a foam roller after eccentric intensive exercise[36]

Should I use the foam roller before or after exercise?

There are benefits for using the foam roller both before and after exercise. Research shows using the foam roller before exercise can increase the range of motion without inhibiting force production. And post-exercise, it speeds up recovery by reducing DOMS.

Denser foam rollers may have a stronger effect than lower density foam rollers. To optimise the benefits from foam rolling, perform 2–5 sets of 30–60 seconds per muscle/muscle group.[37]

---

34 K Nosaka, 'Muscle soreness and damage and the repeated-bout effect', in PM Tiidus, ed., *Skeletal muscle damage and repair*, Champaign IL, Human Kinetics, 2008.

35 (Hill et al., 'Compression garments and recovery from exercise-induced muscle damage: a meta-analysis', *British Journal of Sports Medicine*, vol. 48, no. 18, 2013, pp. 1340–6.

36 AN Schroeder and TM Best, 'Is self-myofascial release an effective pre-exercise and recovery strategy? A literature review', *Current Sports Medicine Reports*, vol. 15, no. 5, 2015, p. 352.

37 Cheatham et al., 'The effects of self-myofascial release using a foam roll or roller massager on joint range of motion, muscle recovery, and performance: a systematic review', *International Journal of Sports Physical Therapy*, vol. 10, no. 6, 2015, pp. 827–38.

THE FTI MOBILITY SEQUENCE

Mobility work is integral to getting clients moving better. Our mobility sequence contains six key facets: warm-up, joint rolling, soft tissue work, mobilisation, activation and stretching.

FTIs approach to mobility

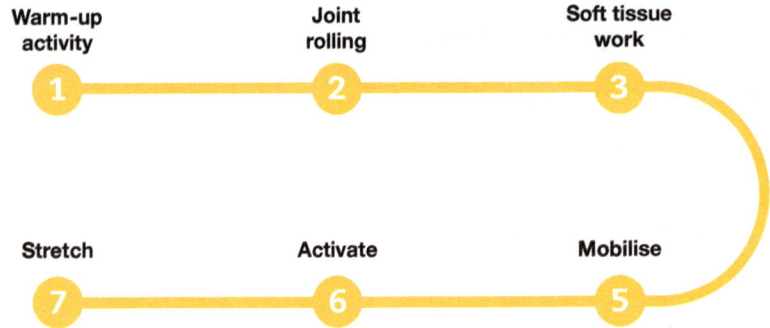

This may be presented as a linear system, but as you gain more experience you will see that sometimes a client needs more focus in one area. They may need lengthening of the muscles, in which case they'll require more and varied stretching in their routine. Or they may benefit from more foam rolling to remove adhesions and tightness in their muscles.

We will now define each element of the sequence. Note that we look at mobilising and activation exercises together in this pillar, as they are closely related in the sequence.

Warm-up activity

A typical training session begins with a warm-up. In traditional programs this may be as simple as getting the client on a treadmill for five to ten minutes, after which they are presumed ready to undertake the program. This kind of warm-up is usually viewed as a necessary evil by both trainer and client.

This is precisely where FTI stepped in to find a smarter way to warm up. In reality, the whole mobility sequence is a warm-up, so we have what we call the 'warm-up activity'. The purpose of this activity is to increase the core temperature of the body, making it more pliable for the next stage of warm-up, which is joint mobility.

This activity to raise body temperature can be done on a bike or rowing machine or through running or skipping. It should take three to five minutes.

Joint rolling

Joint rolling takes old warm-ups and puts them into a system which covers the whole body. It is a gentle way of actively moving joints through a full range of motion (ROM) in preparation for the rigours of exercising.

We recommend clients perform approximately eight rotations of each main body joint in each direction. It should only take three minutes to cover the whole body and leave it warm and pliable for the main workout.

The following set of pictures provides an example of joint rolling the ankle from a more active and balance-challenging postion.

Movement Execution
- 'Draw' five circles clockwise and five circles anti-clockwise.
- Focus your eyes on the horizon as opposed to the foot. This enhances the visual side of training and gives a clear point of focus.
- The tempo needs to be slow, smooth and mindfully performed.

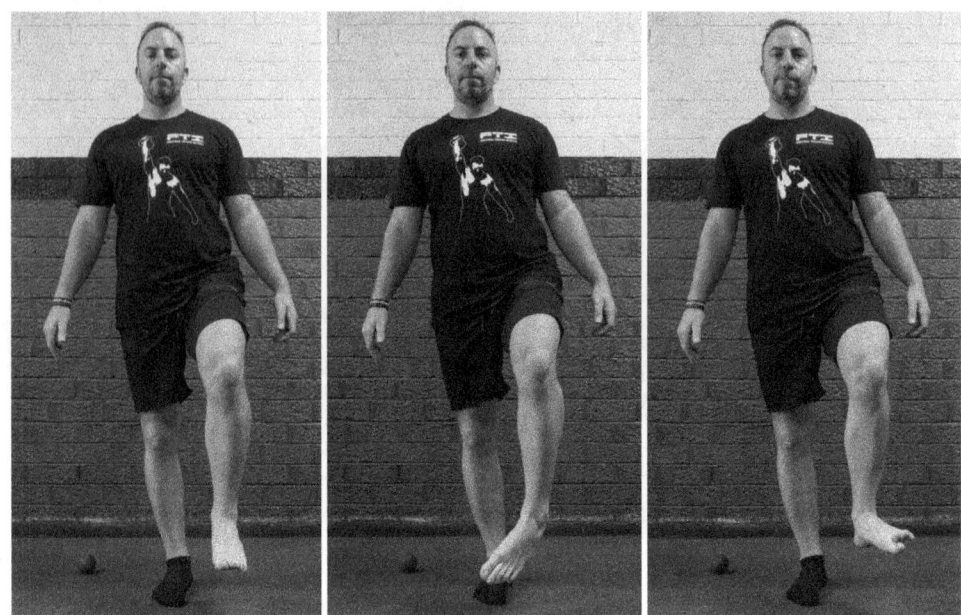

Soft tissue work

Soft tissue or release work is a strategy used to free up 'mechanical knots' found in the belly of the muscle. Soft tissue work can be performed with implements like balls and foam rollers or through passive treatment, as with a remedial massage therapist.

Our simple method is to use a foam roller in what is often termed 'self-myofascial release work'. This can be an empowering way to get clients to take ownership and become autonomous – hence the 'self' element of the term.

Our recommendation to coaches is to select the 'big three' muscles your client needs to work on. Their goal is to roll the length of the muscle from origin to insertion eight to ten times. When clients find a sore spot along the fibres of the muscle belly, they should stop and take a few deep breaths, placing as much bearable pressure on the spot as they can handle.

Note: Get your client to use the RPE scale (rate of perceived exertion from 1–10, where 1 is mild and 10 is extreme). This is a great way to get realtime feedback and build tolerance when performing foam rolling techniques.

The key is to work at a 5–6 on the RPE. Encourage your client to breathe through the process of rolling up and down the muscle.

Duration: Three minutes when performed correctly.

ONLINE RESOURCE: To see more, visit our resource link – http://functionaltraininginstitute.com/book-resources/

Mobilisations and activations

Mobilisations focus on a key joint, functioning to increase the range of movement (ROM) for that joint. It is equivalent to lubricating the joint to alleviate joint stiffness, thereby increasing the range of movement of that joint. At FTI, we follow a 'joint by joint' approach to mobilisations. We need to appreciate and look after the parts before we can work as a whole unit. Each joint has particular needs, as the following table indicates:

Joint by joint approach

Joint	Primary need
Ankle	Mobility (sagittal plane)
Knee	Stability
Hip	Mobility (multi planar)
Lumbar Spine	Stability
Thoracic Spine	Mobility
Scapulo-thoracic	Stability/mobility
Gleno-humeral	Mobility

Activations, sometimes coupled with mobilisations, are focused on the muscles that act on the joint to optimise efficient and safe movement. When key muscles such as the gluteus medius are underactive, we seek to 'switch on' these muscles through activating them.

There are seven key areas that often lack a combination of mobilisation and activation.

The 7 lacking movements

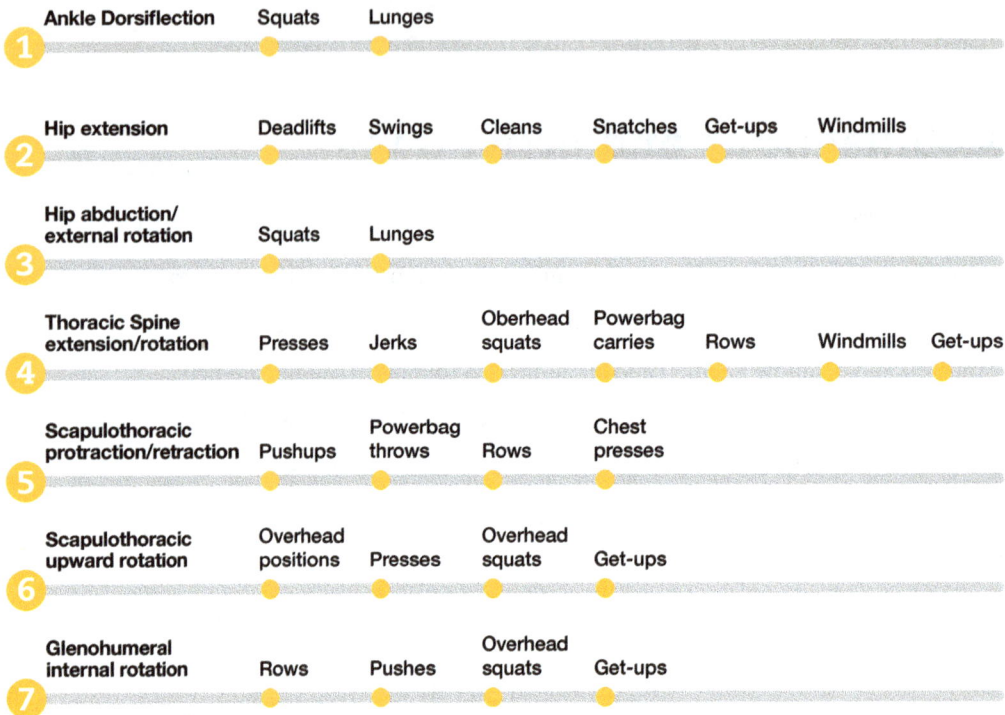

The following section of Pillar 1 charts the seven lacking movements in more detail, showing how to address them through some or all of the following:

- A mobiliser or activation technique
- A release (soft tissue)
- A key stretch
- A functional test

1. ANKLE DORSIFLEXION

Mobiliser – Wall drill

Movement Execution

- Find and face a wall
- Place one foot in front and step the other back
- Place your hands on the wall and keep the foot of the front leg flat
- Slowly draw the knee to the wall while keeping the foot strictly flat
- Once the foot starts to shift (e.g. heel raising or foot collapsing inward), measure the distance of the big toe to the wall. The optimal distance is 7.6 cm from the wall to your foot.

Note: Take shoes off for a more accurate measure. Test the other foot and see if there is a significant difference, which may compromise functional movements like squats and lunges.

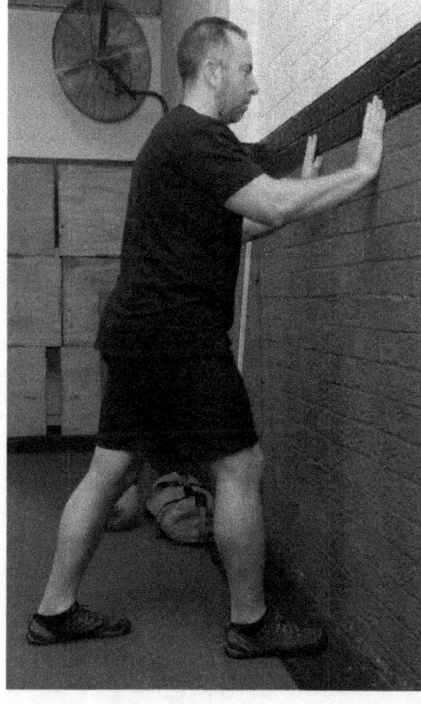 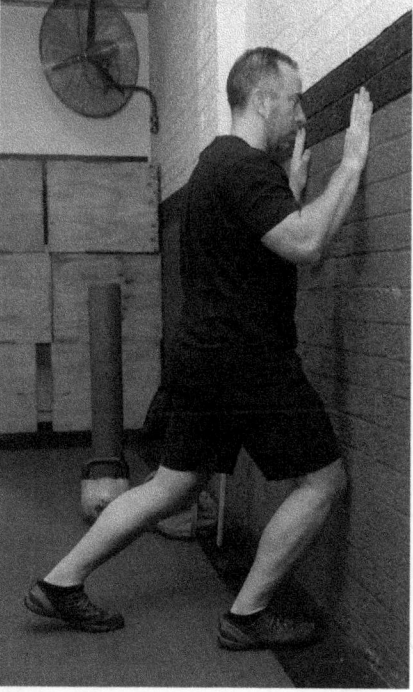

Active release – Calf foam rolling

Movement Execution

- Start with both legs on the foam roller
- Hands are flat to the side and trunk is upright
- Slowly roll from origin to insertion of the calf (see pictures 1 and 2)
- Note: to advance this, simply place one foot on top of the other and focus on placing adequate pressure as you move up and down on that particular calf (pictures 1 and 2)

Note: Remember to hold the areas where there is a knot and pace adequate pressure for 15-20 seconds.

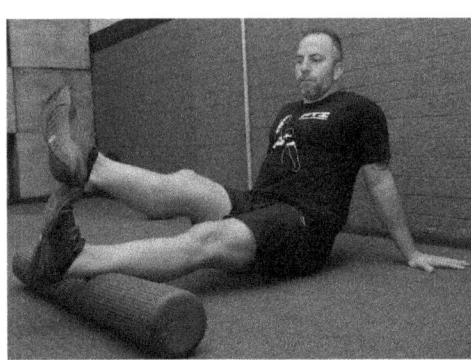
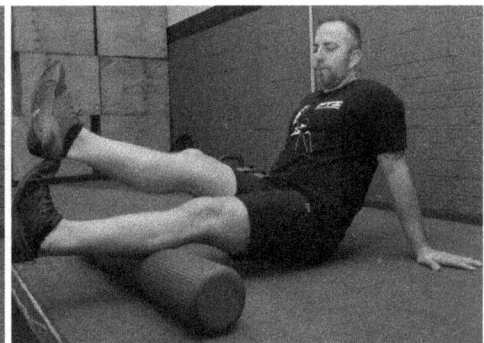

Functional test – Squat

After completing the ankle mobiliser and active release, get the client to perform a few bodyweight squats to see how they are moving. Ask them how it feels as they move through the motion 3–5 times. Give specific and simple feedback.

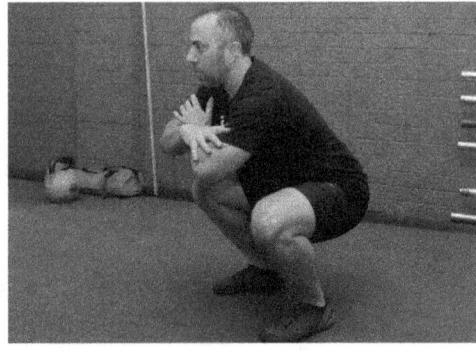

2. HIP EXTENSION

Mobiliser – Lunge hip pulse

Movement Execution

- In a lunge position with back knee cushioned as an option, flex the hip of back leg (picture 1)
- Extend the hip and hold for 3 seconds (picture 2)
- Release back into flexion and perform again

Note: Perform 5 on each leg. Make sure you breathe in as you pulse the hip into extension, then breathe out as you go into flexion.

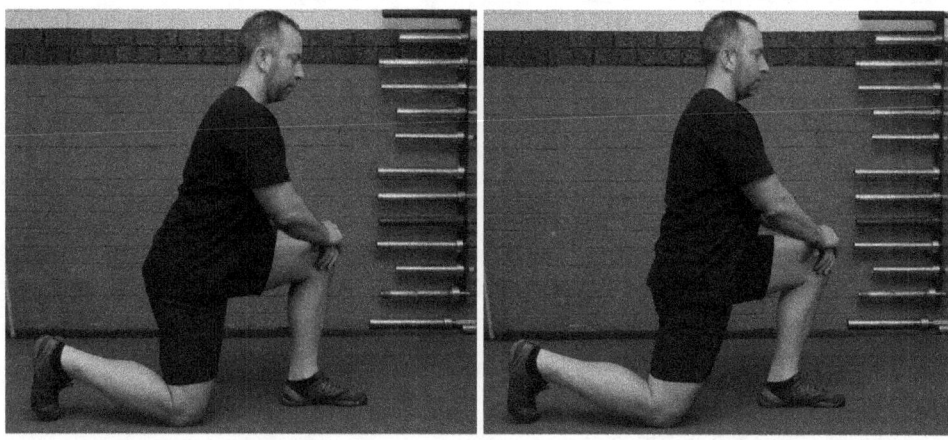

Release – TFL release

Movement Execution

- There are two tool options for this release: a kettlebell handle or a mobility/trigger ball
- Place the kettlebell handle or trigger ball into the TFL
- Place adequate pressure for 10–15 seconds at a time
- Shift the ball or kettlebell handle slightly side to side to get the full area of the TFL
- You can also use a wall with the ball to offset the extreme pressure some people may feel when performing it with these two particular options

Note: The TFL feels like a rounded chunky muscle and goes to the greater trochanter. The TFL can be palpated by using an internal rotation of the hip – a rounded bit of tissue will pop up.

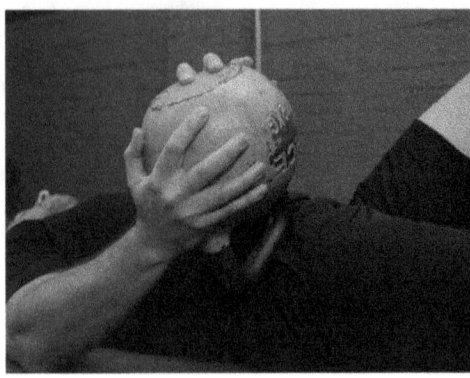 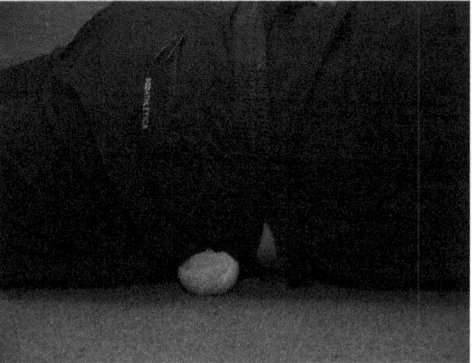

Activation – Glute bridges

Movement Execution

- Lying flat on your back, tuck the heels close to your bottom. Fan out the knees and the toes (picture 1)
- Slowly drive the hips toward the ceiling, assuming full extension for 3 seconds (picture 2)
- Slowly lower to the floor
- Repeat 5–8 times or as desired

Note: Having hands flat to the sides is a regression and having the hands pointing toward the ceiling (as in picture 2) is an advanced option.

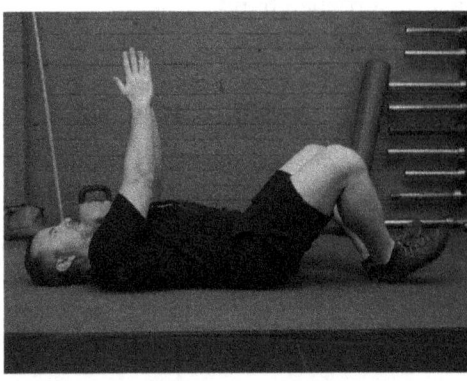 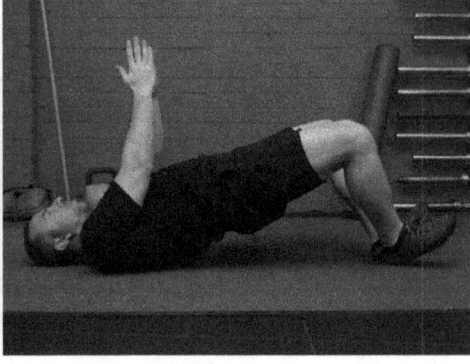

Functional test – Kettlebell Romanian deadlift

After completing the hip extension mobiliser, release and activation, get the client to perform a few Romanian deadlifts to see how they are moving. Ask them how it feels as they move through the motion 3–5 times. Give specific and simple feedback.

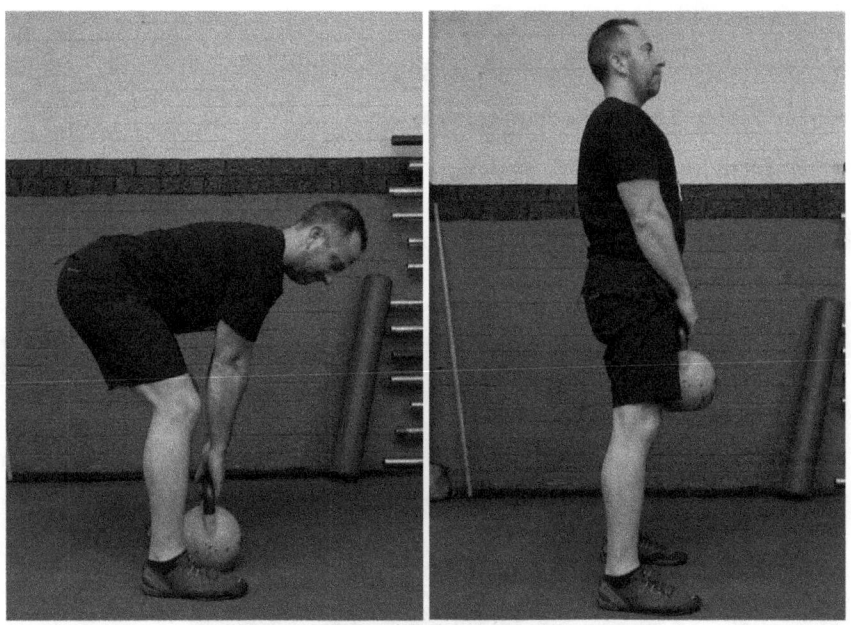

3. HIP ABDUCTION/EXTERNAL ROTATION

Mobiliser – Half goblet squat hold

Movement Execution

- Have feet wider than a usual squat
- Push the hips toward the wall and keep trunk in a strong neutral position (picture 1)
- Wedge the elbows inside the thighs and gently push the knees out
- Hold for 3–5 seconds, then release
- Perform for 5–8 reps or as desired

Note: Ensure you do not drop too low into the position. This is not intended as a deep squat.

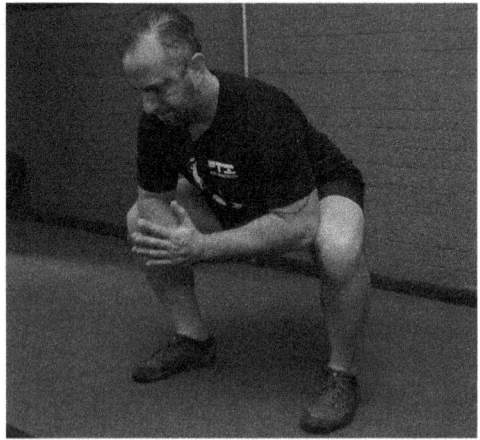

Release – Adductor foam rolling

Movement Execution

- Assume the position (picture 1)
- Keep spine straight and ensure the lower back does not sag
- Slowly roll across the adductors into the insertion area (picture 2)
- Perform 5–8 times each leg

Note: Work at different angles as you roll from one end to the other.

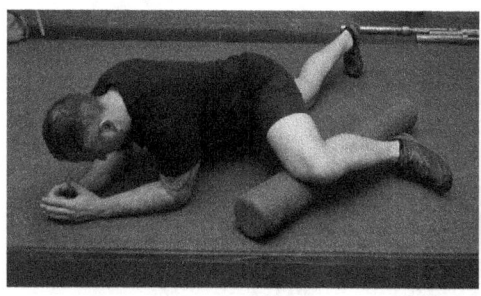 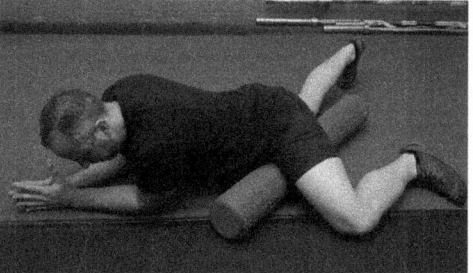

Functional test – Cossack lunge

After completing the mobiliser and release, get the client to perform a few Cossack lunges to see how they are moving. Ask them how it feels as they move through the motion 3–5 times. Give specific and simple feedback.

Movement Execution

- Choose a kettlebell and assume an upright position (picture 1)
- Lunge across to one side ensuring you do not collapse the trunk (picture 2)
- Work to the best range you can and then drive back up to standing
- Perform on the other leg
- Perform 2–3 reps each leg or as desired

Note: To hit the Adductor 'flexor group' (Brevis, longus and gracilis) rotate the foot inward so that the knee will now point forward.

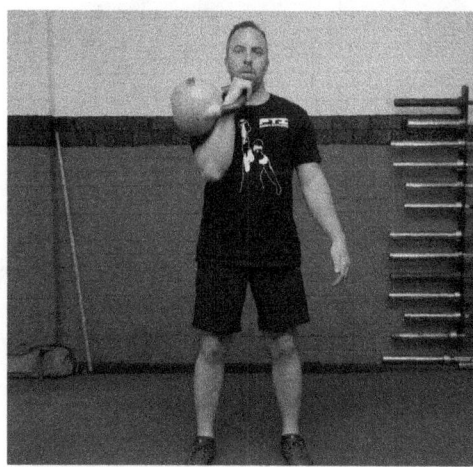 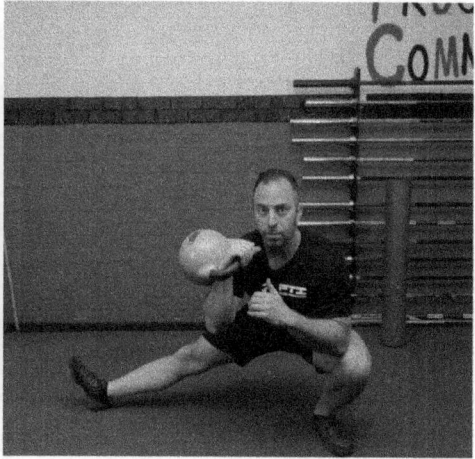

4. THORACIC SPINE EXTENSION/ROTATION

Mobiliser 1 – T-spine foam rolling

Movement Execution

- Place foam roller at the bottom border of the scapula
- Place hands behind head and draw elbows in (picture 1)
- Take a breath, and as you breathe out extend the back (picture 2)
- Perform 5–8 times or as desired

Note: Try to go gradually deeper into the movement.

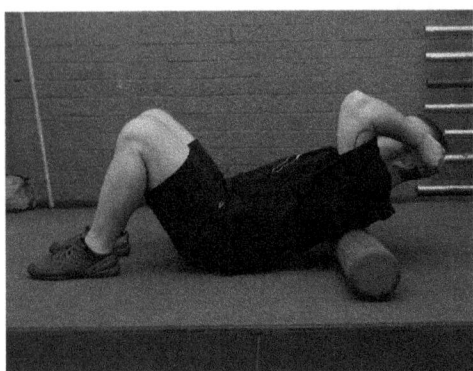 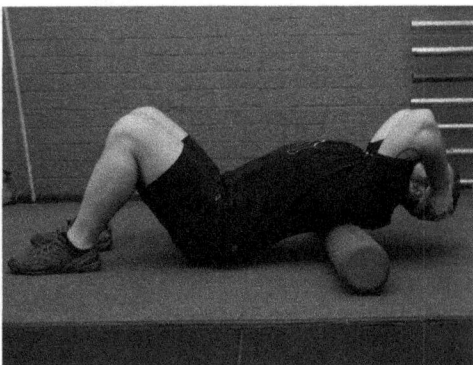

Mobiliser 2 – Quadruped extension/flexion drill

Movement Execution

- Assume a quadruped position (all fours contacting the ground)
- Take one hand and place it on the back of the head
- Draw the elbow toward the opposite arm, which remains extended (picture 1)
- Slowly open up the chest and draw the elbow toward the ceiling (picture 2)
- Perform 5 times on each side or as desired

Note: Do not force the movement (picture 2). Gradually increase the rotation and extension that this wonderful mobiliser offers.

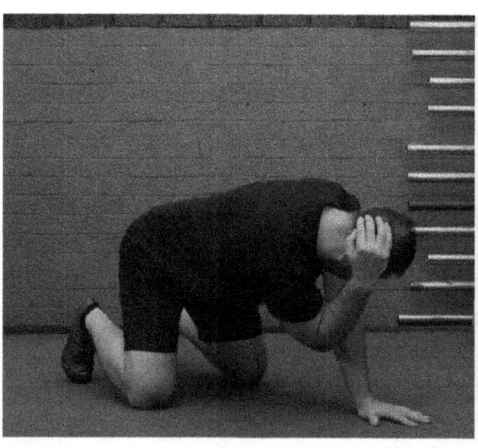 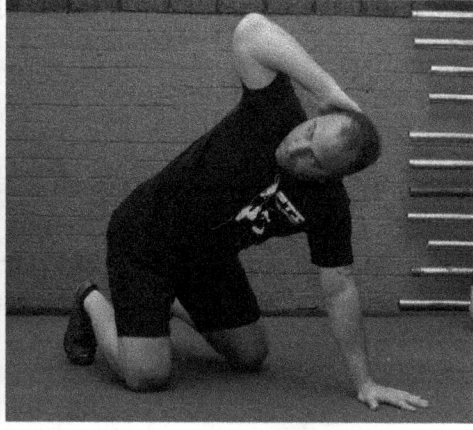

Activation drill – Standing T rotations

Movement Execution

- Assume a hip hinge position with hands in front (picture 1)
- Slowly rotate as far as you can without compensating through the lower back (picture 2)
- Slowly come back to the start position and perform to the other side (picture 3)
- Perform 5 times to each side or as desired

Note: Remember to perform the movement in a slow and controlled manner.

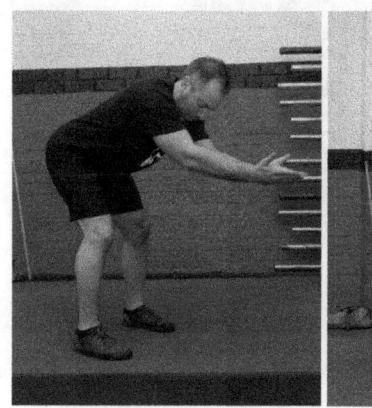 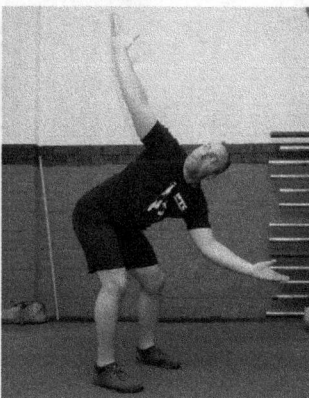 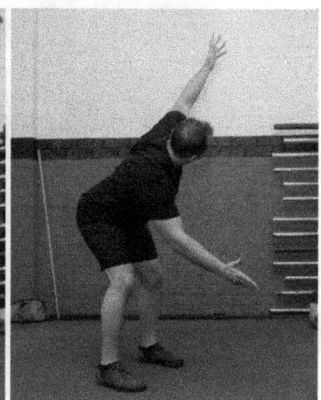

Functional test – Rotational deadlift

After completing the mobiliser, release and activation, get the client to perform a few rotational deadlifts to see how they are moving. Ask them how it feels as they move through the motion 3–5 times. Give specific and simple feedback.

Note: Start with a lighter weight and elevate the weight to make the movement easy enough so that it is a test and not part of a workout.

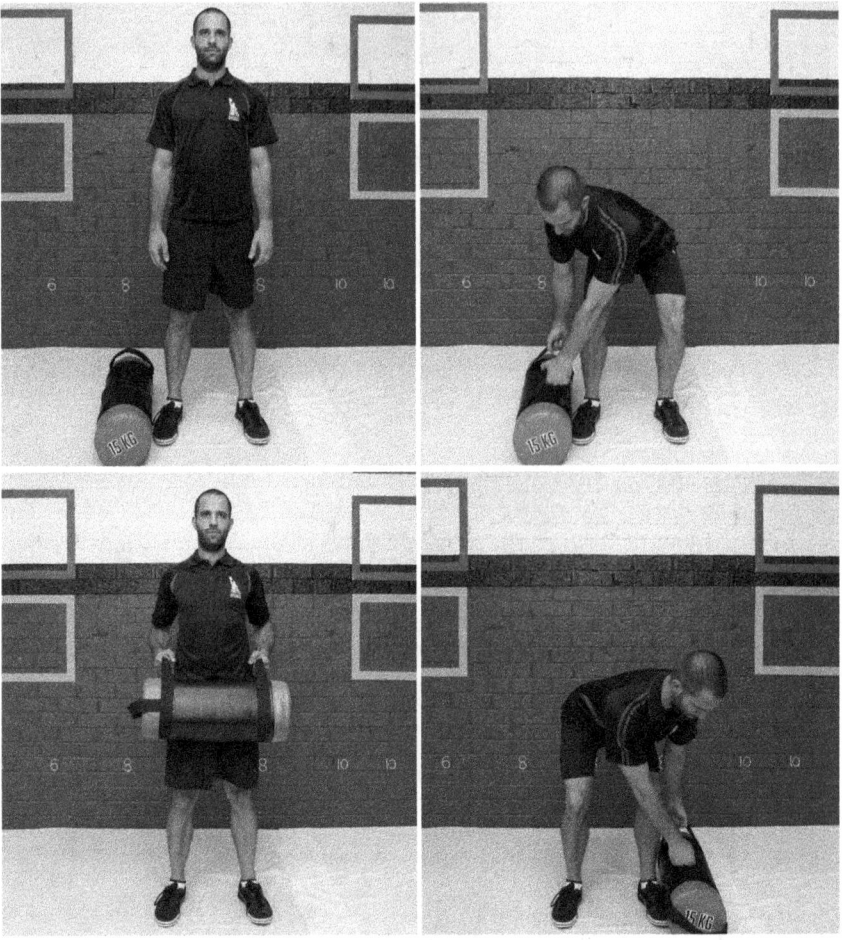

5. SCAPULOTHORACIC PROTRACTION/RETRACTION

Mobiliser – Standing arm swings

Movement Execution

- Protraction phase: in a standing position, cross the arms, keeping elbows in line with shoulders (picture 1)

- Retraction phase: Swing the arms back in a controlled manner (picture 2)

- Perform 5–8 times

Note: Each time you cross the arms into protraction, cross them over alternately. This will add a further coordination element to the movement.

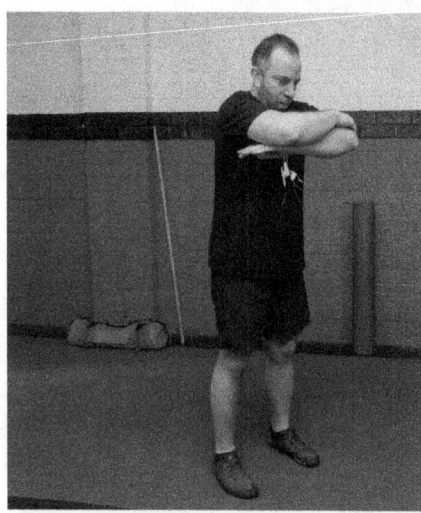 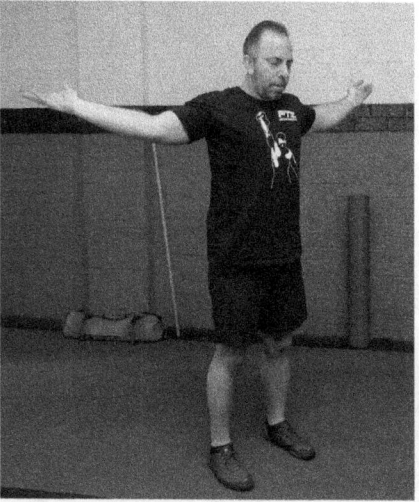

Activation drill – Scap push-up

Movement Execution

- Assume a high plank position as though you are ready to perform a push-up (picture 1)
- Push the ground away, keeping elbows locked'
- Squeeze the scapular together, focusing on the top half of the back (picture 2)
- Perform 5–8 times or as desired

Note: This is a tricky movement to get at first. We advise adopting a kneeling position and practising the protraction (picture 1) and retraction (picture 2) of the movement first (see pictures 3 and 4).

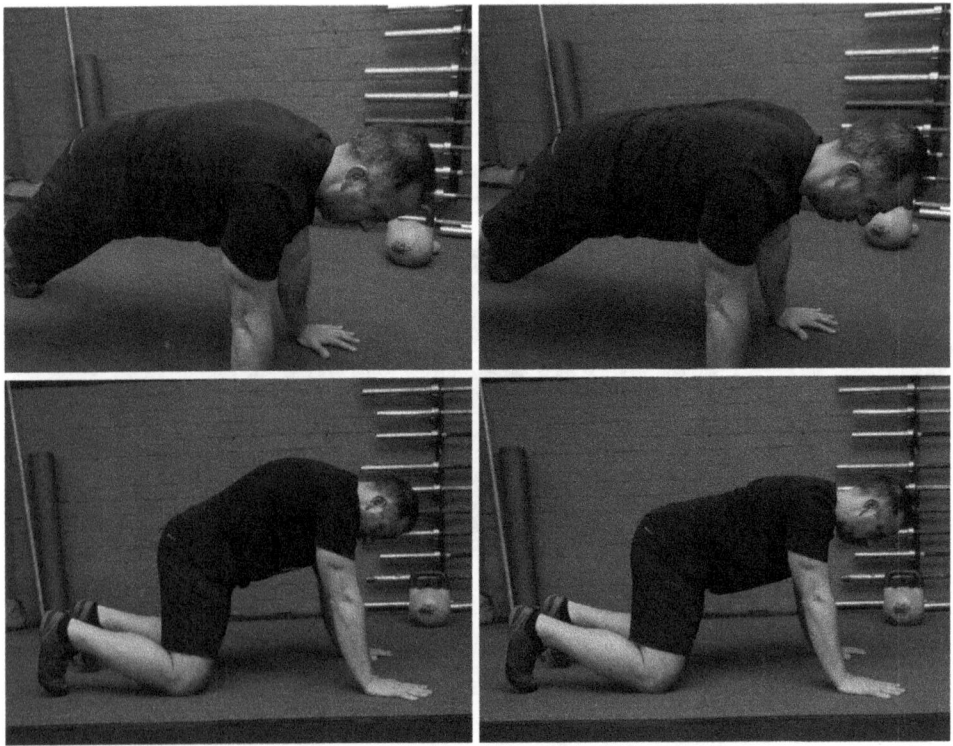

Functional test – Upright suspended fitness push-up

After completing the mobiliser and activation, get the client to perform the upright suspended fitness push-up to see how they are moving. Ask them how it feels as they move through the motion 3–5 times. Give specific and simple feedback.

Note: Observe how the scapula is moving throughout and ensure the push-up is performed in a controlled and slower manner, not rushed.

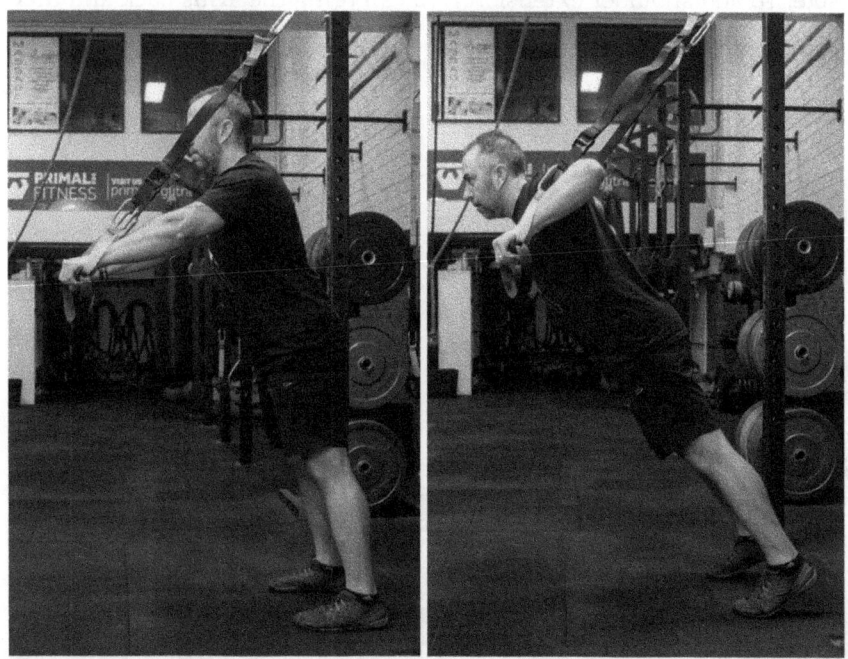

6. UPWARD ROTATION

Mobiliser 1 – Standing sagittal arm swings

Movement Execution

- Keep arms to side in a standing position (picture 1)
- Swing the arms up without arching through the back (picture 2)
- Repeat 5–8 times or as desired

Note: To add shoulder extension, you can bring the arms back and then swing them to an overhead position (shoulder flexion).

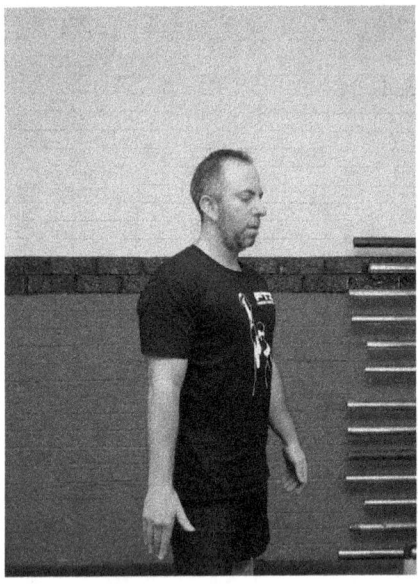 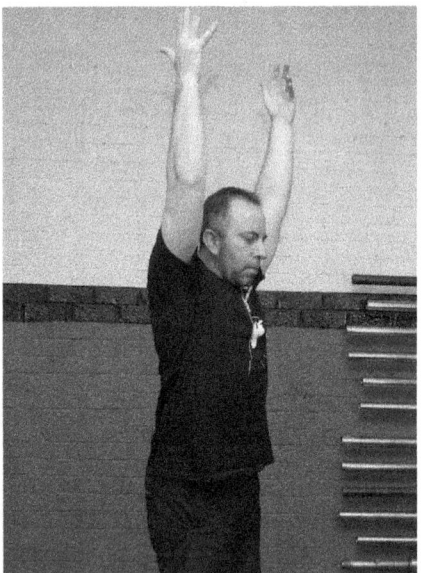

Mobiliser 2 – Wall slides

Movement Execution

- Stand against a solid wall with elbows at 90 degrees and flat to wall (picture 1)
- Slowly draw the arms up without completely locking them overhead (picture 2)
- Perform 5–8 times or as desired

Note: The avoidance of locking out is to ensure maximum activation of the scapula in upward rotation. Make sure your heels are slightly off the wall to increase the activation of the movement.

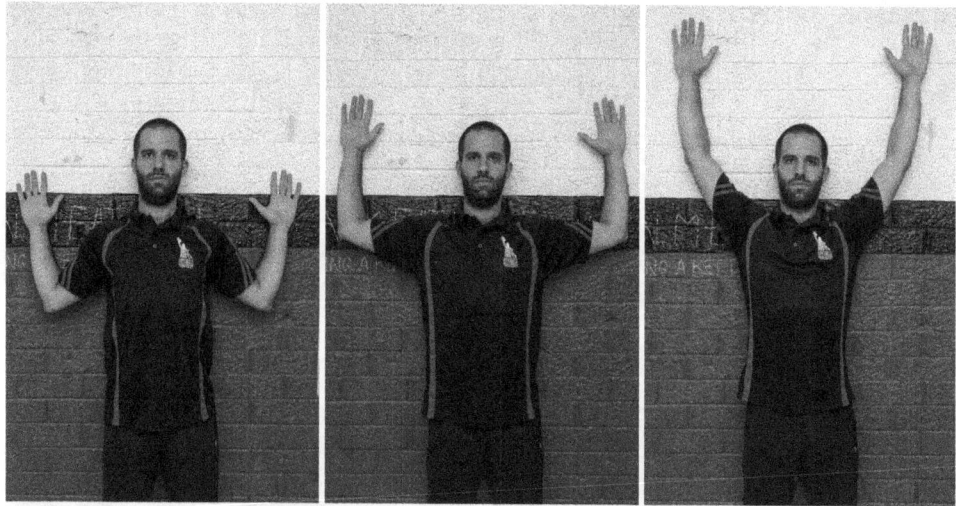

Release drill – External rotators/lat foam roll release

Movement Execution

- Lie on a foam roller with the hand cradling the neck to the side you are working on (picture 1)
- Roll back and forth across the external rotators and partly into the lat (picture 2)
- Perform in a controlled and slow manner 5–8 times each side

Note: Breathe through the movement and try to relax into it.

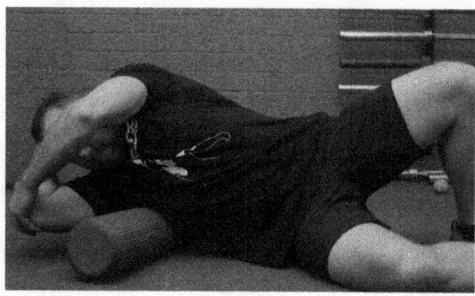
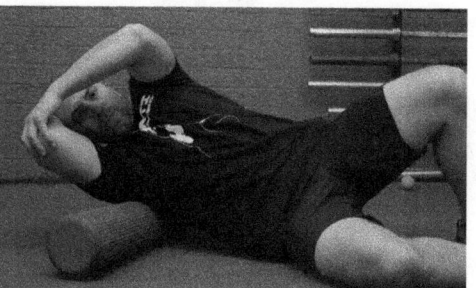

Active stretch – Lat mobiliser

Movement Execution

- Reach across with the arm you are working on and place the other hand on top to lock it in (picture 1)
- Take a breath and move into the stretch as you breathe out (picture 2)
- Come back to position 1 and perform the movement again
- Perform 5 times on each side

Note: Keep the working arm as extended as possible to get more of a lat stretch.

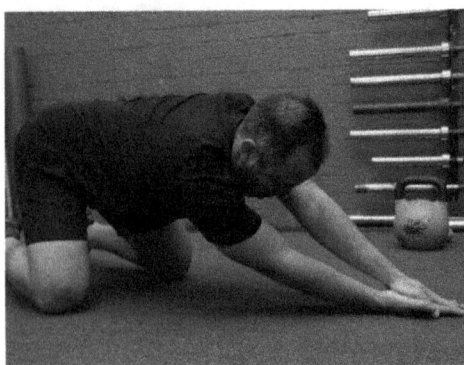 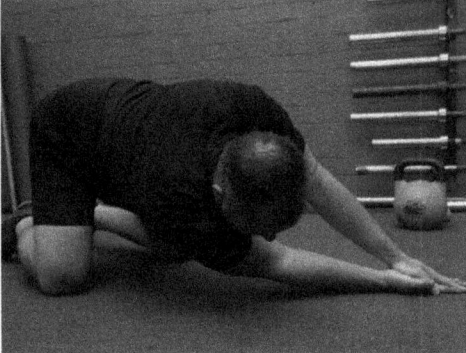

Functional test – Standing kettlebell press

After completing the mobiliser and release, get the client to perform the overhead kettlebell press to see how they are moving. Ask them how it feels as they move through the motion 3–5 times. Give specific and simple feedback.

Note: Perform a few reps to each arm in a controlled manner. Observe what is happening to the scapula and if compensations are taking place.

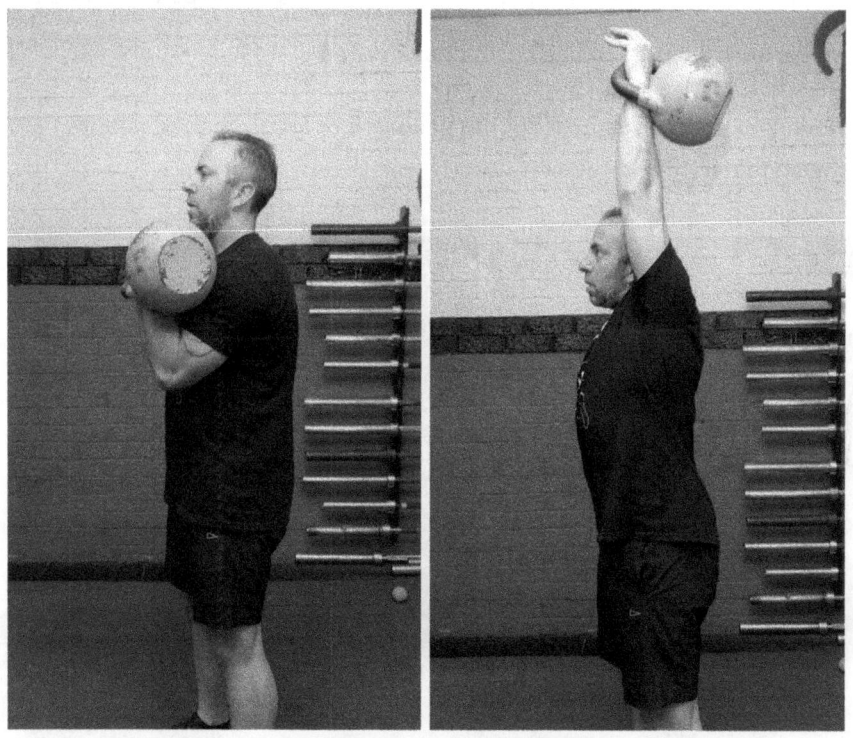

7. INTERNAL ROTATION

Mobiliser – Standing suspended fitness trainer test

Movement Execution

- Loop the arm into a set of straps and keep the elbow level with the shoulder (picture 1)
- Keep the shoulder packed, then rotate the arm inwards with the other hand supporting (picture 2)
- Perform in a controlled manner and do not push the pain threshold
- Perform 5 times on each arm or as desired

Note: You may have one side that you need to focus on to rebalance the shoulder.

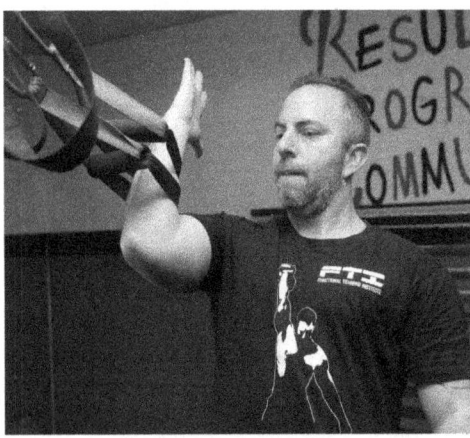
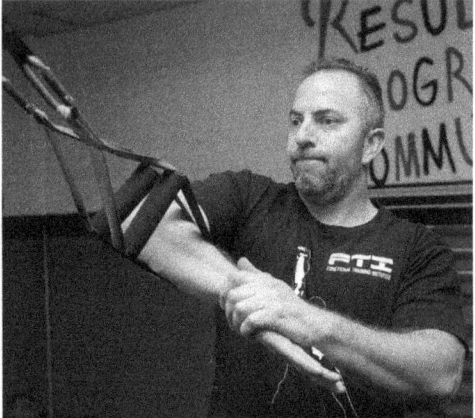

Release – Pec minor drill

Movement Execution

- Take a trigger ball (a lacrosse ball is great) and place it into the groove of the chest (picture 1)
- Sink the ball into the area, targeting the pec minor as you do so
- Draw the ball across and under the clavicle (neck area) to the front of the shoulder

- Find a wall and perform the movement slowly (picture 2)
- Hold the tight spot for 20 seconds then release, keeping the opposite arm extended to the side
- Perform 5 times on each side or as desired

Note: Learn to feel the area shown in picture 1. This will stimulate the fascia and ensure you perform the movement correctly.

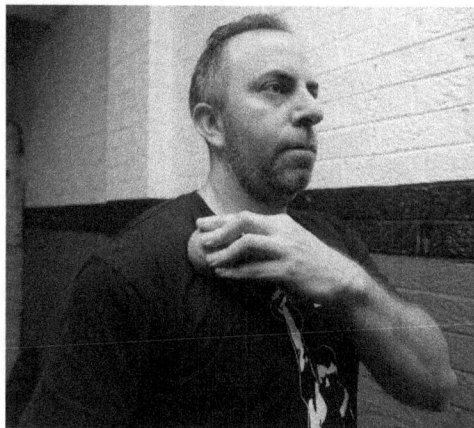 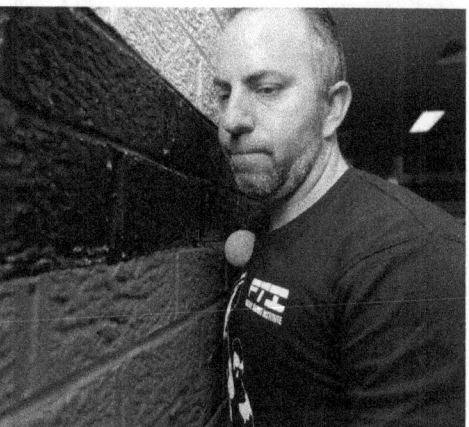

Activation – banded press drill

Movement Execution

- Take a piece of physio tubing and tie it to a pole or have someone be the anchor (picture 1)
- Make sure the arm is 45 degrees to the side and there is sufficient pressure from behind
- Slowly raise the arm up in a controlled manner and slowly bring it down to the start position again (picture 2)
- Perform 5 reps on each side

Note: The tubing should not be too strong. This technique ensures the serratus anterior and subscapularis (two muscles that are underactive during pushing movements) are recruited.

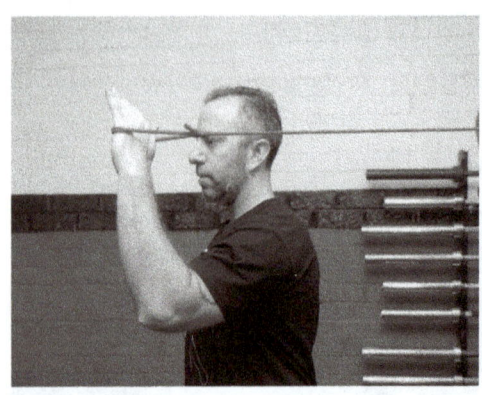
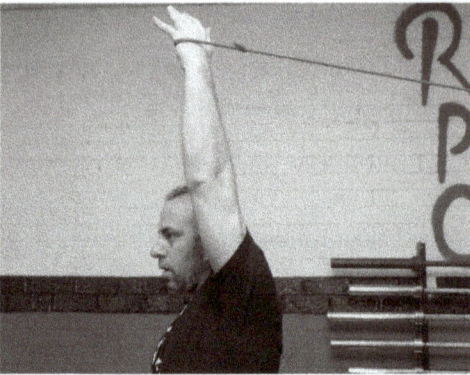

Functional test – Lying kettlebell chest press

After completing the mobiliser, release and activation, get the client to perform the lying chest press to see how they are moving. Ask them how it feels as they move through the motion 3–5 times. Give specific and simple feedback.

Movement Execution

- Lying flat on the back, safety roll and keep the kettlebell in a neutral position (picture 1)
- Keep the back flat and slowly draw the kettlebell toward the ceiling (picture 2)
- Perform 3 on each side

Note: You need to be familiar with the safety roll to perform the movement.

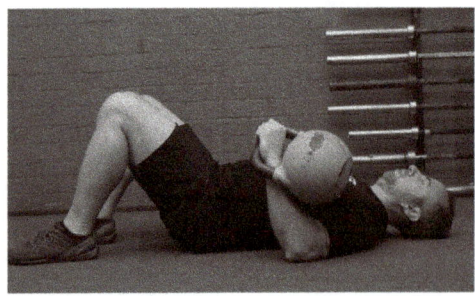
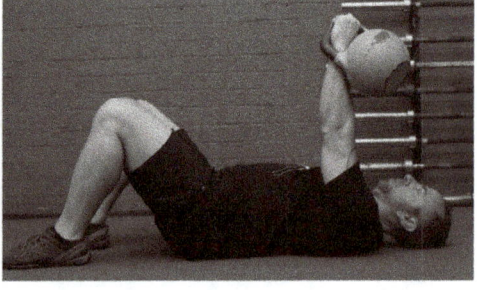

ONLINE RESOURCE: To watch the lying chest press video, go to our resource link – http://functionaltraininginstitute.com/book-resources/

Stretching

Muscle tension is inversely related to length. When muscle tension is increased, muscle length is decreased. Conversely, when muscle tension is decreased, muscle length is increased. Therefore, to improve flexibility muscle tension must be decreased.

As part of a flexibility training program, stretching is used to increase the distance between a muscle's insertion and origin. There are three main types of stretching:

STATIC STRETCHING

- Static stretching involves holding a joint in a specific position, then holding this position at the end of range with the muscle on tension to a point of a stretching sensation.

- Static stretching prior to exercise has been shown to decrease strength and power by approximately 5–30%.[38]

- The loss of strength resulting from acute static stretching has been termed 'stretch-induced strength loss'.

- Static stretching may assist with muscle recovery and therefore is most beneficial after exercise.

DYNAMIC STRETCHING

- Dynamic stretching involves moving a limb through its full range of motion to the end ranges and repeating several times.

- Dynamic stretching is the most beneficial type of stretching to engage in prior to strength and explosive-based exercises.

- Dynamic stretching is not associated with strength or performance deficits, and actually has been shown to improve jumping and running performance.

---

38 (Young 2002).

PNF (PRE-CONTRACTION) STRETCHING

- PNF is performed by having the client contract the muscle being used during the technique at 75–100% of maximal contraction, holding for ten seconds, and then relaxing. Resistance can be provided by a partner or with an elastic band or strap.

- PNF stretching is often used in rehabilitation programs; however, PNF stretching is also considered an advanced form of stretching that may be more effective for intermediate to advanced gains in flexibility.

- PNF stretching is best undertaken after exercise.

For best 'bang for buck' when integrating stretching, choose 'the big three' exercises we outline here, which are a combination of active and passive PNF-based stretches.

PNF Stretch 1 – Pec minor

This is a great PNF stretch to do before or after a session.

Movement Execution
- Have client lie along a foam roller
- Place heel of palm on the crest at each end of the pec
- Get client to press shoulder blades back and take a breath in
- Slowly press down on their pecs and get client to breathe out slowly
- Release and repeat 5 times, or to your desired effect

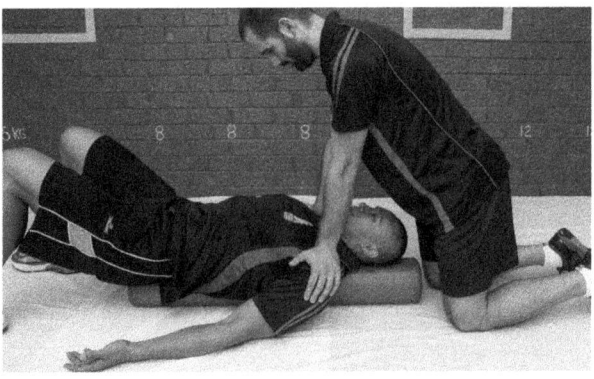

PNF Stretch 2 – Hip flexor

This is a tremendous technique to lengthen those tight hip flexors.

Movement Execution

- Get client to lie on a bench or foam roller
- Client hugs one knee to the chest, keeping back flat
- Lightly push down on the opposite hip flexor
- Ensure client breathes in and out
- Release and repeat 5 times, or to your desired effect

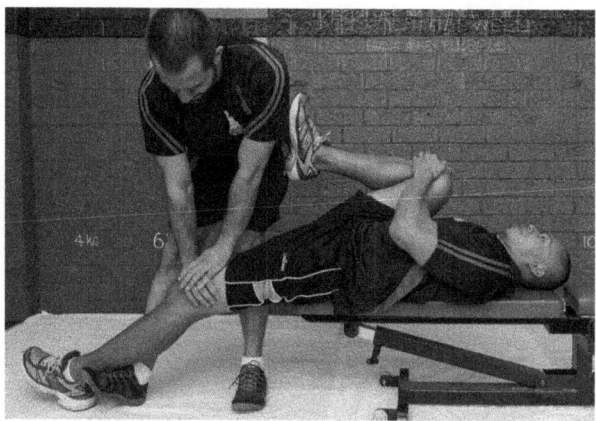

PNF Stretch 3 – Thoracic spine

This can be done on your own without assistance from another person

Movement Execution

- Use a bench or an object of similar height and sturdiness
- Hold dowel in supine position (palms facing up)
- Peg elbows to the edge of the bench
- Breath in and, as you breathe out, sink down between the arms
- Lengthen the back as much as possible as you work deeper into the stretch
- Perform 3–5 reps

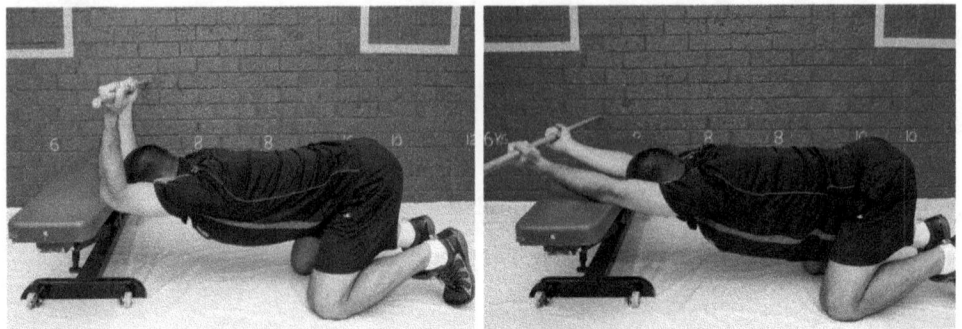

Mobility flows and movement prep

As we move our clients along the dysfunction to optimal movement continuum, it is essential to appreciate that in order to integrate, we need to isolate and work on the weaknesses that our client has. However, we then need to reintegrate.

In his insightful book *Movement*, Gray Cook describes a 'parts versus the whole' approach to the body, noting that 'patterns and sequences remain the preferred mode of operation in biological organisms'. Cook paints a clear and useful picture of how personal trainers and functional fitness coaches may consider this in our own profession:

'Viewing the parts can give clarity but viewing the patterns will produce a global understanding. Studying the details imparts movement intelligence, but understanding the patterns creates movement wisdom.'[39]

As we understand from classical anatomy, nerves innervate muscle and the central nervous system sends electrical and chemical signals to perform an action under a sympathetic or parasympathetic response. What this means for us and our clients is that we want to decrease stress and trauma and cultivate an environment conducive for optimal movement.

By taking into consideration not just muscular but neural imbalances, we can look into strategies that will help us consider coordination and neural

---

39   Gray Cook, *Movement: Functional Movement Systems*, Aptos CA, On Target Publications, 2010, p. 8.

training to facilitate better movement. Such strategies have become more prominent in recent times, popularised by programs like Mike Fitch's Animal Flow® and Tim Anderson's Original Strength.[40] The premise behind Original Strength is that we have lost the naturally healthy patterns of movement we had as a toddler/young child and we can regain optimal movement via a series of 'progressive resets'.

ONLINE RESOURCE: To view Original Strength resets video go to – http://functionaltraininginstitute.com/book-resources/

Drawing from the wisdom of these approaches, we encourage coaches to incorporate flows into their programs. Flows are bodyweight-based and can be used in conjunction with the isolated methods we have covered thus far. Once you have understood the basics of the Adaptive FTS Mobility Sequence, you can take a more integrated approach that considers mobilisers and activations in a series of simple to more complex flows and movement preparation.

Mobility flows have many benefits:

- You can create a series of specific movements for your client or group. The specificity principle applies as much to a warm-up as it does to the main guts of the workout.

- Flows can be made easier or harder. Adding more complexity requires some thought and will depend on the fitness level of your client.

- Flows bring in greater levels of neural control, stability and skill work which is all part of having your client move with quality and not simply quantity.

- In using flows, you reduce the risk of injury. The last thing we want is to create an environment where the risk factor is increased due to lack of an effective and smart warm-up.

40   www.animalflow.com, www.originalstrength.net

- You can treat flows as a screening process before the main workout. By making this part of the warm-up challenging enough, you can ensure your clients are not at risk when performing the main workout.

In Pillar 1, the key is to keep flows simple. They are more about movement preparation than 'doing a workout'. More strenuous flow applications are part of Pillar 2.

We've included a great flow here called 'Scorpion progression'. Our friend and international partner Joey Alvarado from KettleJitsu is the genius behind this flow. It is best done in three parts, as outlined in the following pictures.

Try this sequence five times through and it will provide a great way to integrate mobilisers and activations with an emphasis on skill.

PART 1 – SCORPION TAPS

Movement Execution

- Lie flat on belly with arms wide like a cross (picture 1)
- Slowly rotate one leg to reach toward the opposite hand (picture 2)
- Do not overextend yourself at this point
- Gradually increase the range as you warm into it
- Perform on the other side (picture 3)

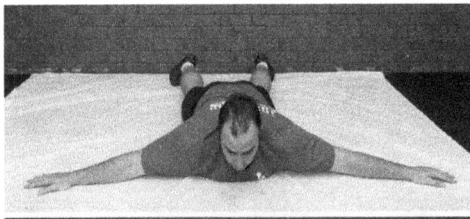
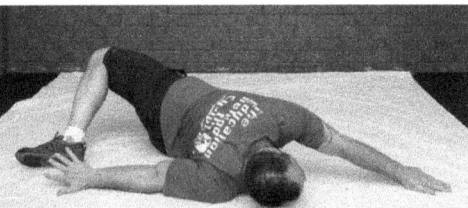
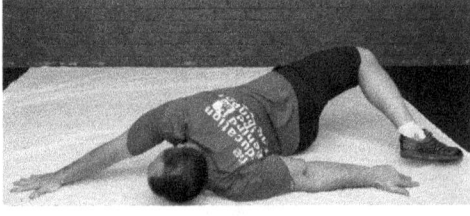

PART 2 – SCORPION ROTATIONS

Movement Execution

- Keep hands close to chest, then push away from the ground (picture 1)
- Using momentum, swivel to the opposite side (pictures 2 and 3)
- Smoothly come back to start position and perform on other side (pictures 4, 5, 6)

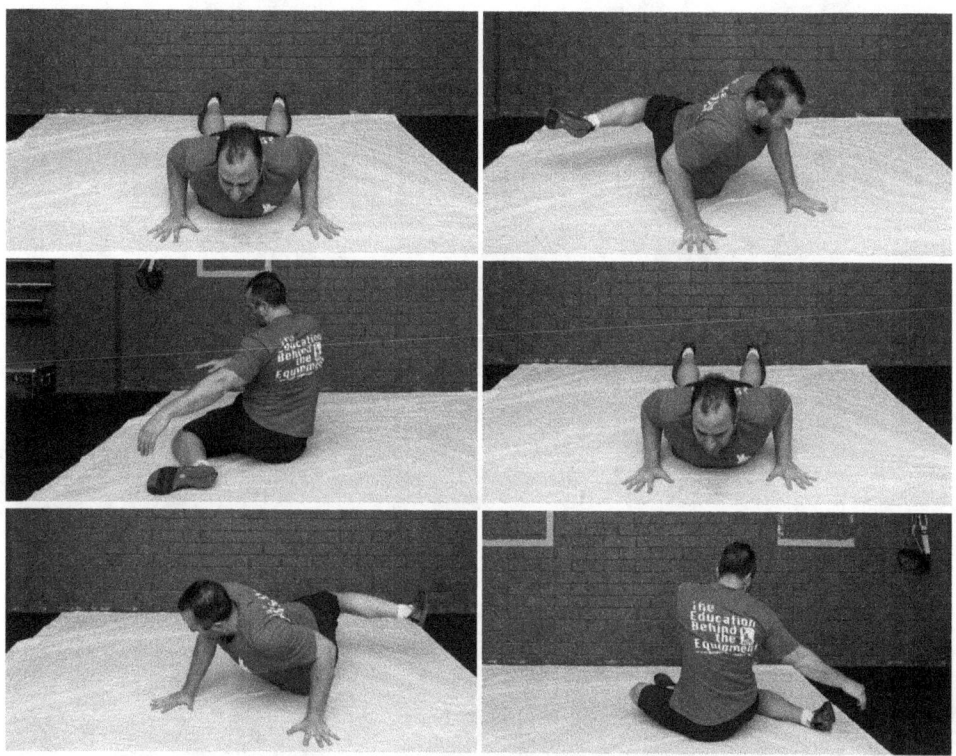

PART 3 – SCORPION BRIDGE

Movement Execution

- Push away from the ground (picture 1)
- As you swivel around plant one hand behind (picture 2)
- Pop the hips up into a bridge, reaching with the other hand to the ceiling/sky (picture 3)
- Slowly lower and perform on the other side (pictures 4, 5, 6)

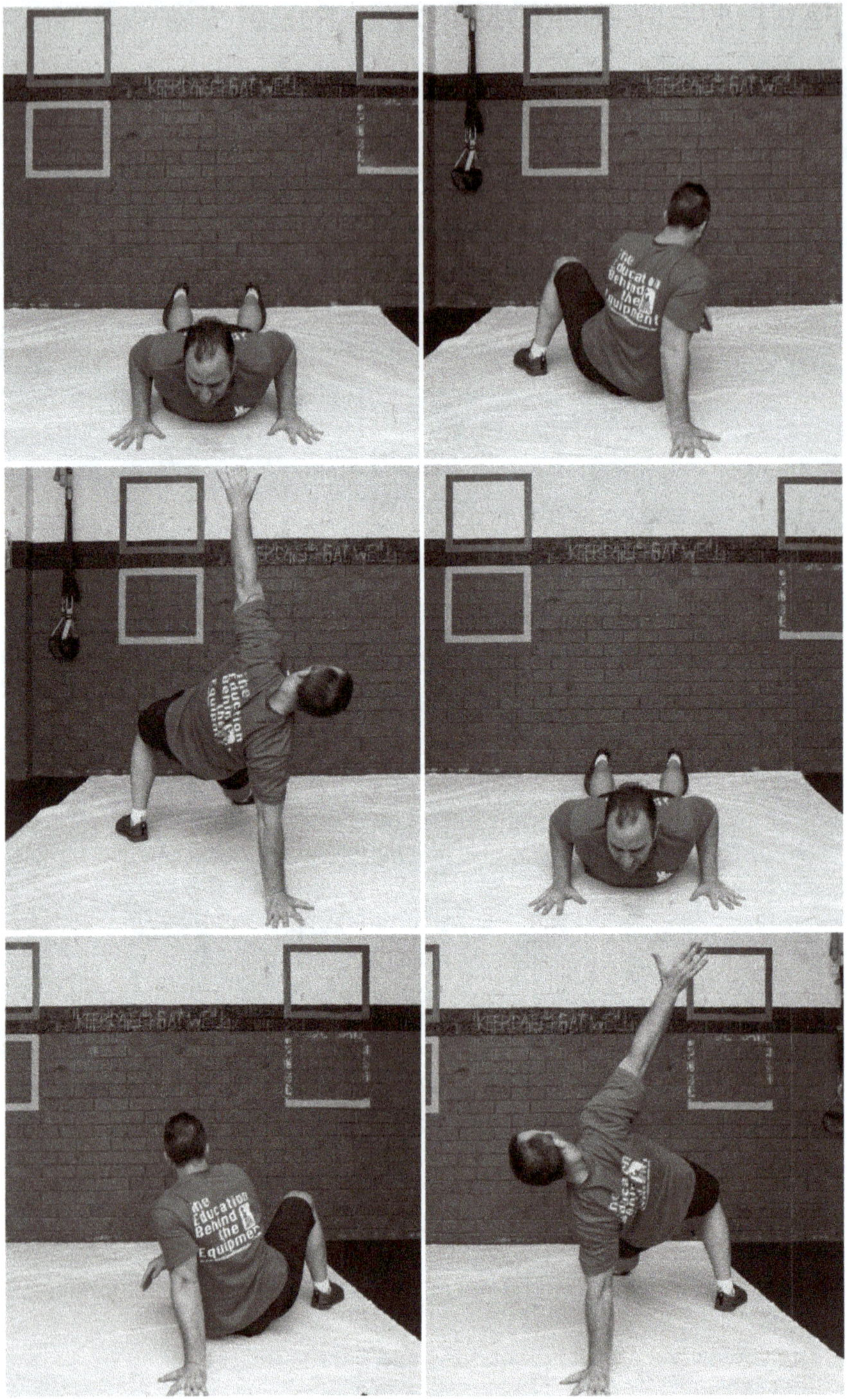

 ONLINE RESOURCE: To view flows in action, visit our resource link – http://functionaltraininginstitute.com/book-resources/

160   PURPOSE DRIVEN MOVEMENT

Recap

In this chapter we have covered the six stages of FTI's mobility sequence, with a primary focus on explaining and demonstrating the activation and mobilisation movements. Performing mobility is not just a task a coach does to warm up clients. It is part of our broader commitment to healthy movement and ongoing biomechanical and injury screening.

When coaching mobility, we need to be specific with the mobiliser and activations we introduce, which will form the movement preparation portion of the program or workout. We must also consider the importance of introducing mobility flows to bring together the various mobiliser and activation strategies, as this will increase client coordination and neural preparedness.

Restoring function and movement is the important first step before moving on to the next pillars. Mobility is not something the coach leaves behind when a client begins to move better. It will always form part of a smart workout and is the functional movement bedrock from which we can now explore the next pillar in the Adaptive FTS.

Pillar 2 – Develop Proper Movement Patterns

We have a saying at FTI: 'If they can't do it, don't load it.'

Where there is a culture driven by image and the need to be strong, there is a method flawed with a lack of understanding and intelligent application. There are trainers out there who feel the need to always add load, even where there is clear movement dysfunction. By loading clients who have no strength foundation coupled with poor gross movement patterns, such coaches are creating more dysfunction and inevitable chronic injury and pain. This is the opposite of what we want to achieve. It compromises the efficacy of screening and program, not to mention the trust between coach and client that is an essential part of growing toward optimal movement.

Our focus in Pillar 2 is therefore to explore bodyweight movement prior to loading. This pillar builds on the function and movement restoration of Pillar 1, focusing on advanced crawling and neural patterns to develop greater bodily awareness, leading into more pattern-specific movements. As Gray Cook states, 'Patterns are groups of singular movements linked in the brain like a single chunk of information. This chunk essentially resembles a mental motor program, the software that governs movement patterns.'[41]

At FTI, we believe that the key to a successful program lies in progression and variety. If a client cannot do a loaded squat, in what ways can we create a continuum and at what stage do we start them in their journey? By creating a pathway to progression, we instil in the client a sense of achievement. It is 'earning the right', their right, to movement mastery.

---

41   Gray Cook, *Movement: Functional Movement Systems*, Aptos CA, On Target Publications, 2010, p. 8.

In this pillar we look at the role bodyweight training plays in movement progression and performance. To understand one's own body and how it feels when performing movement is the most important element of bodyweight training.

So, what is bodyweight training? If I were to ask a hundred movement coaches what bodyweight training means to them, I may well get a hundred definitions.

Bodyweight training expert and founder of the CrankIt suspended fitness training method, Owen Bowling, defines it this way:[42]

- Bodyweight training is about movement. Movement is a fundamental human need that serves to enrich our experience of our own body and the world around us. Anyone that has experienced a restriction of their ability to move, whether through injury or circumstance, knows how much this impacts their quality of experience.

- Bodyweight training is both a means to an end and an end in itself. By incorporating bodyweight movement training you can improve a variety of physical and mental attributes as you work toward a specific goal of health, fitness or physique. But you also reap the benefits of movement for movement's sake, which is a powerful end result in its own right.

- When applied correctly to a holistic exercise program, bodyweight training will serve to build a solid foundation of coordination and movement mastery, which can then be applied to other forms of exercise.

In the first part of this pillar we look at some of the theory behind bodyweight training: the importance of the body's sling systems, primal movement patterns and the benefits of barefoot training. We then look at two bodyweight training applications: suspended fitness and Animal Flow®.

---

[42] From an email exchange between author and Owen Bowling. See www.crankitfitness.com

Bodyweight movement: sling systems and primal patterns

The body is a complex system made up of anatomy slings, which are comprised of muscles, fascia and ligaments all working together to create stability and mobility. When the anatomical slings are balanced, they produce efficient movement, force and speed.

The concept of myofascial slings comes out of the work done by researchers like Andy Vleeming, Diane Lee and Thomas Myers, whose textbooks illustrate the many fascial connections within the body.[43] The theory of myofascial slings states that the body is connected by certain fascial lines which enhance how muscles work together to create a movement.

When a muscle contracts, it produces a force that spreads beyond its attachment points. When balanced, these forces are then transmitted through the muscle-fascial connections within the anatomical sling, providing optimal alignment of the musculoskeletal system during dynamic movement. Four important anatomical sling systems work together for load transfer through the pelvic/lumbar region. These are:

- **The anterior oblique sling:** The anterior oblique system (AOS) consists of the external oblique and internal oblique, connecting with contralateral adductor muscles via the adductor-abdominal fascia. When this group of muscles contract together, they increase lumbopelvic stability.

- **The posterior oblique sling:** This sling system consists of the latissimus dorsi (LD), the gluteus maximus (GM), and the interconnecting thoracolumbar fascia (TLF). The posterior oblique sling plays an important role in the control of movements such as human gait.

- **The lateral sling:** The anatomy of the lateral sling consists of the gluteus medius, gluteus minimus, tensor fascia latae (TFL) and iliotibial band

---

43 Andy Vleeming, 'The thoracolumbar fascia', *Fascia: The Tensional Network of the Human Body*, Robert Schleip et al., London, Elsevier, 2012, p. 37; Diane Lee, *The Pelvic Girdle E-Book: An Integration of Clinical Expertise and Research*, London, Elsevier, 2012; Thomas Myers, *Anatomy Trains E-Book: Myofascial Meridians for Manual and Movement Therapists*, London, Elsevier, 2013.

(ITB). The lateral sling is used in frontal plane stability and controls pelvic stability in dynamic movements such as gait, lunges and stair climbing.

- **The deep longitudinal sling:** The deep longitudinal sling connects the erector spinae, multifidus, thoracolumbar facia, sacrotuberous ligament and the biceps femoris. This sling allows for movement in the sagittal plane while simultaneously influencing local stability.

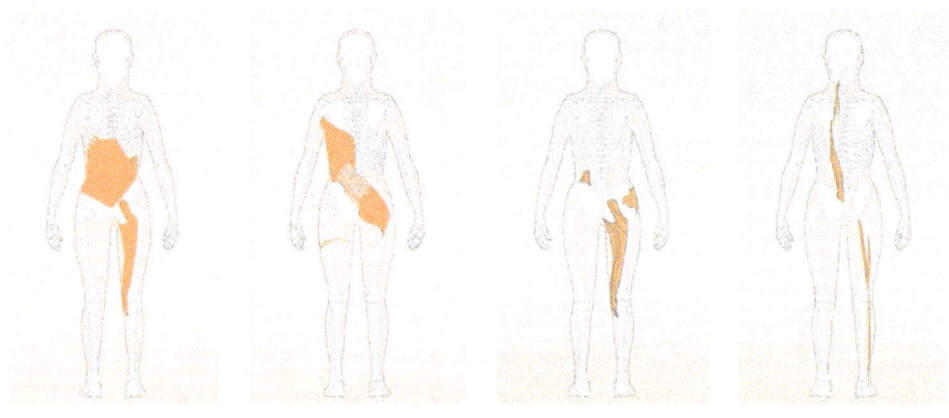

The anterior oblique sling   *The posterior oblique sling*   *The lateral sling*   *The deep longitudinal sling*

Understanding the sling system in relation to movement enhances our ability to design programs that are not simply rotational in nature. By incorporating the sling system into functional movement, we create greater lumbo-pelvic stability, which in turn helps us to create greater power when performing movements and exercise programs.

The slings can be loaded just as effectively in bodyweight training as in loaded training. Think of the movement produced in simply walking. Both the anterior and posterior sling systems work together to allow the pelvis to initiate the contralateral movement of the swinging arm and opposing swinging leg during movement. It is essential to understand how the sling systems are used in basic movements like this before entering into loaded movement training.

This is where the 'primal movement patterns' come in.

SEVEN PRIMAL MOVEMENTS

Primal movements are patterns of moving that are fundamental to us all but get lost in our sedentary lifestyles. In his legendary book titled *How to Eat, Move and Be Healthy*, Paul Chek elaborated on seven primal movement patterns that have served the human race for thousands of years.[44]

As we have learned in the coaching foundations, there is no better way to communicate a movement to clients than creating a story or analogy that will invoke an instant recognition of what you're teaching them. Here are some of the ways we get clients to recognise the primal movements in their daily lives:

1. **Push:** Imagine your car has stalled on the side of the road and you and your buddy are left wondering what to do. You get outside and within a reasonable distance there is your beacon of hope: a petrol station! Instinctively you get behind the boot, side by side, and begin to *push* the car toward the petrol station. Life is full of daily scenarios where we must push against something. Have any of us thought about the effect of gravity and how if we orient our body in certain positions, we can leverage this gift of nature? Some of us curse a push-up – yet how fundamental a building block this movement is for bodyweight application.

2. **Pull:** Most Australian households have a lawn mower, or at least have seen one before. Functionally speaking, they are great for getting our butts off the couch and performing a movement that involves walking and pushing, coupled with changing angles to get those tricky bits of grass cut. To get the engine started so you can cut the grass, we must *pull* the cord, sometimes only once but, if you're like me, two or three times before it gets going.

---

44 Paul Chek, *How to Eat, Move and Be Healthy*, Vista, CHEK Institute, 2004.

- **Twist:** Have you ever had the inconvenience of placing something in the back seat of the car and having to *twist* to retrieve it? It is such a familiar and instinctive thing to do. Hopefully your car was stationary at the time and your back is still intact.

- **Bend:** You are taking a lovely stroll on a sunny Sunday morning when suddenly you notice your shoelaces are undone, almost causing you to trip over. With a roll of the eyes, you *bend* down to tie up the laces. Let's hope no one was behind you!

- **Squat:** Ever been to a country that requires you to truly and deeply *squat* to do your business? Enough said.

- **Lunge:** You are playing touch footy with your children and their friends in the local park. Things are going swimmingly until, out of desperation, you *lunge* to try to make contact with your child (who goes on to score without being stopped).

- **Crawl/walk/run:** You are watching your baby crawl and you get so inspired you begin crawling with your baby in a 'crawl train'. You notice that your baby is so much smoother and proficient at it than you.

These examples illustrate daily functional movement for us, and no doubt you can think of other scenarios and activities that match these primal patterns.

When we couple an understanding of the anatomical sling systems with the primal movement patterns, we begin to build a clear picture of the movements that need to be rehearsed and refined in bodyweight training prior to loading.

One further thing to consider before embarking on bodyweight sequences is the important role of the feet in training.

STAYING GROUNDED IN BODYWEIGHT TRAINING

Whenever we are performing movement, with or without load, we are adding a compressive force. Quite simply, gravity is a compressive force we are constantly resisting in order to function in our daily lives. Equally important is the interplay between compression and tension.

If we look at a tensegrity structure (see the tensegrity model), we can see that the rods are held in a system of tension – in this case, elastic banding. If we compress one rod and collapse it inward, then it will affect the entire structure.

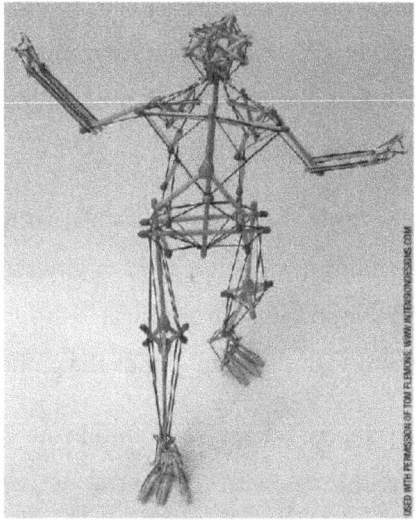

Similarly, our body is held together by a network of fascia that allows us to transmit force in tandem with our joints and muscles. As we have already explored with the sling systems, force transmission requires a coordinated effort that is affected from the ground up. Proper alignment and loading of the joints will ensure a reduction in injury and greater force production due to stable and mobile joints.

If we look at the distribution of power from the ground up, we know the feet play an essential role here. Dr Emily Splichal, podiatrist and global leader in barefoot education, elaborates on this further:[45]

- When it comes to the concept of dynamic force production or the transfer of ground reaction forces the human foot and our body's relationship to the ground is often times the missing link in human performance.

- Often overlooked and taken for granted, foot function and its association to the rate of neuromuscular stabilisation is deeply seated in the evolution of human movement. As the only contact point between the body and the ground, the foot must be appreciated as a powerful neuromuscular structure and what I truly believe to be the 'gateway to the nervous system'. Acting as our base or our foundation, any instability or delay in stabilisation of the foot-ground relationship will immediately translate proximally into the hips and pelvis.

- The skin on the bottom of the foot is packed with powerful proprioceptors or nerve endings, which respond to different stimulation. This plantar proprioceptive stimulation is critical to the way in which the foot – and therefore the nervous system – reads the ground.

- Adjusting to every step we take or every shift in our centre of gravity, the plantar foot communicates with the central nervous system, creating a neuromuscular response between our feet and our centre of gravity or the core. Proprioceptive stimulation of the foot leads to a reflexive contracture of the intrinsic or small muscles of the foot. These intrinsic muscles of the foot are fascially connected to the deep muscles of the core via the deep front fascial line. I refer to this as foot-to-core stabilisation, and it is the foundation to human movement.

- This foot-to-core pathway is fed through the sensory stimulation of the plantar proprioceptors. Any damping of these plantar proprio-

---

45   Emily Splichal, www.emilysplichal.com. This material was provided to FTI directly.

ceptors by shoes, orthotics and certain surfaces creates a delay in our body's stabilisation. This delay in stabilisation eventually leads to compensated movement patterns, inefficient movement and an increased injury risk.

The most effective ways to optimise foot-to-core stabilisation is through barefoot stimulation, training on smarter surfaces and integrating minimal footwear.

- Barefoot stimulation does not mean do not ever train with shoes on. Integrating at least five minutes of purposeful barefoot movement prep at the start of your client's or athlete's sessions is a good start. Consider integrating trigger point release as well; five minutes applied to the bottom of the foot yields an immediate improvement in postural control.

- Opt for training surfaces that naturally vibrate such as wood, grass, dirt or any suspended flooring. Our nervous system receives increased proprioceptive information from surfaces that vibrate. Surfaces to avoid include concrete, rubber, sand and marble.

- Footwear must be considered, as cushioning in shoes blocks the proprioceptors of the feet resulting in instability, altered reaction time and an atrophy of the intrinsic muscles of the feet. Ideal footwear for proper foot-to-core stabilisation is minimal cushion, minimal heel-toe drop and no midsole in the shoe. This ideal footwear would allow full freedom of movement and maximum control of the ground.

Our call to action as coaches is to help our clients establish healthy pre-loaded movement that gives a pathway to mastering the primary movement patterns. This pre-loaded movement will need to activate the sling systems through primal movements, aided by good foot-to-core stabilisation, thus building 'relative strength' into our clients' programs. We therefore need to focus on the progressions, regressions and variations that will allow us to achieve this objective.

Let us now investigate bodyweight application from two perspectives. The first is the suspended fitness model and the second is Animal Flow®.

Suspended fitness

Suspended fitness is one of the world's most popular functional training methods. At FTI, we work alongside CrankIt Fitness, an Australian company that has created excellent movement-centric suspended fitness techniques.

The reason we have chosen to explore suspended fitness is because the tool provides a comprehensive framework in which to establish initial mastery of one's own bodyweight. Although the application surpasses this in the form of advanced calisthenics, the suspended fitness trainer allows the coach to easily progress and regress a client according to their fitness levels.

The key techniques and exercises that will build up a client's level of coordination, skill and movement efficiency are:

1. Squat
2. Lunge
3. Chest press
4. Pull
5. Hamstring curl

1. SQUAT

Using a suspended fitness tool like the CrankIt Straps or TRX allows users to regress both the load and stability of a bodyweight squat. The specific technique used also promotes engagement of the glutes and can reduce load through the knee joint. This helps beginners and unstable users progress toward mastering a bodyweight squat.

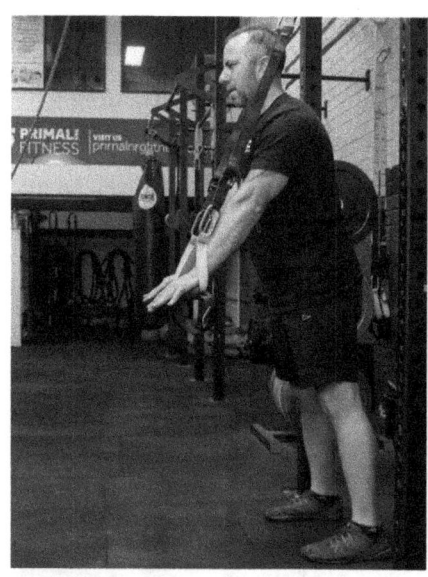 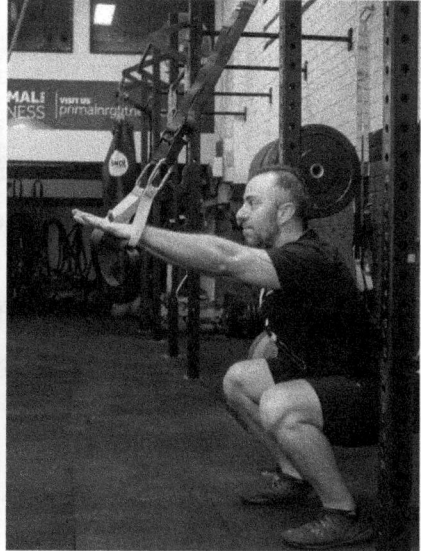

2. LUNGE

The lunge is an exercise that many people do not master prior to adding load. By using a suspended fitness tool, users can engage the lat-glute connection of the back functional line to promote glute activation while also reducing load if required. Once these levels have been mastered, you can progress to a suspended lunge to advance load, stability and complexity.

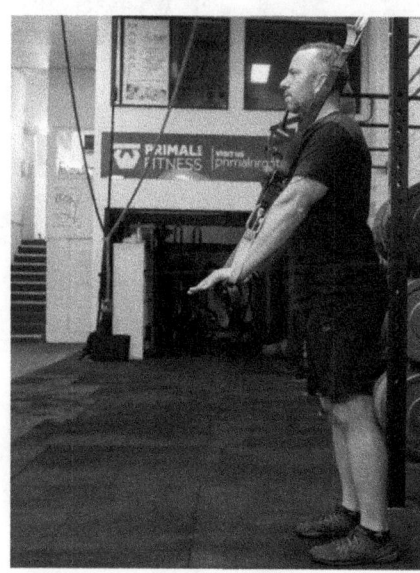 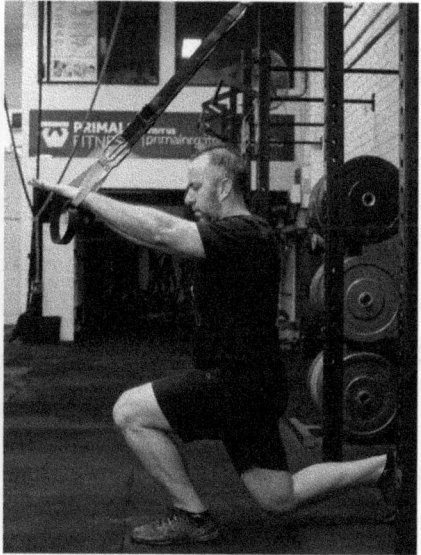

3. CHEST PRESS

The suspended fitness chest press allows for freedom of movement for the scapula, and the load can be easily regressed to allow the user to focus on technique and shoulder function. The instability of the hand-connection point also initiates higher levels of core integration, and the prone position requires a focus on core engagement and neutral spine position. All of these help the user develop transferrable movement and postural skills that will benefit many other exercises they perform.

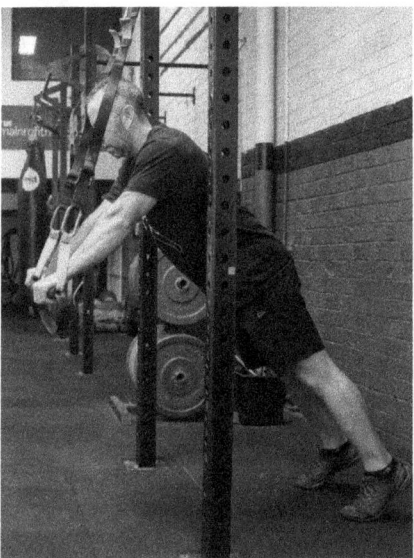
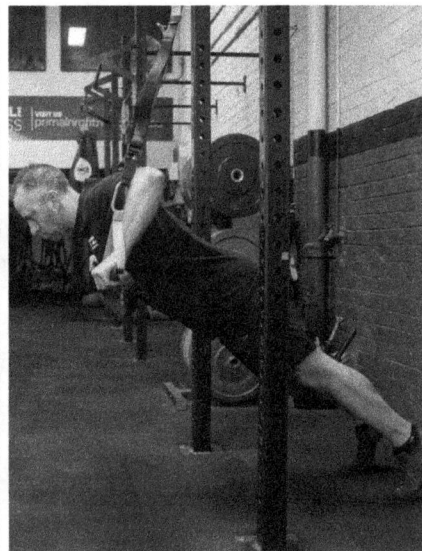

4. PULL

The suspended fitness pull allows for freedom of movement for the scapula, and the load can be easily regressed to allow the user to focus on technique and shoulder function. Users can see and feel for the correct shoulder movement to help avoid the common anterior humeral glide associated with push and pull movements.

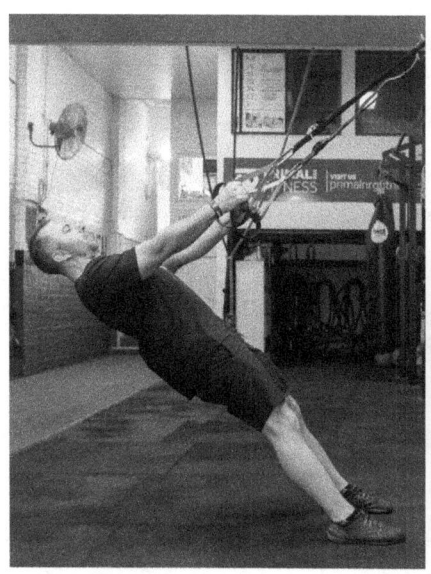 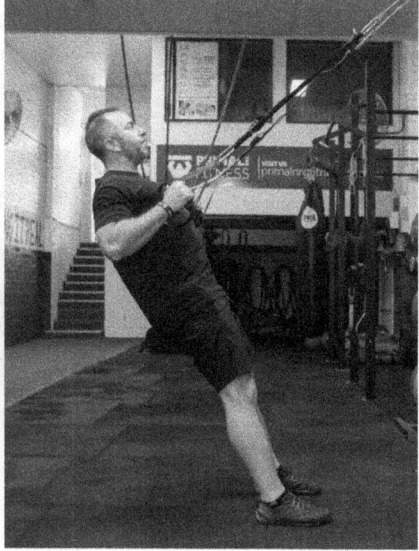

5. HAMSTRING CURL

The specific technique of the suspended hamstring curl promotes the co-contraction of both hamstrings and glutes at the same time. The eccentric focus and instability of this exercise both contribute significantly to reducing hamstring injury risk.

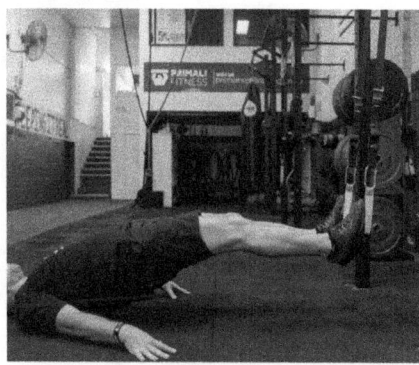 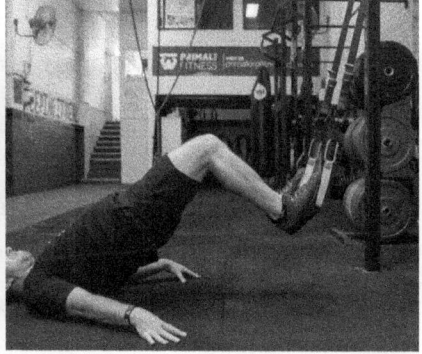

Crawling and Animal Flow®

Building on the bodyweight application, we can explore the methods of progressive groundwork and flows to build a more stable and supple body. One of the most progressive and creative programs to have hit the fitness market is Animal Flow® from Mike Fitch.[46]

The Animal Flow® program combines quadrupedal and ground-based movement with elements from various bodyweight training disciplines including gymnastics, breakdancing, parkour and hand-balancing. The full body, multi-planar movements are great for improving mobility, strength, endurance, power and neuromuscular coordination. The program:

- Is entirely bodyweight training based, using closed-chain exercises to achieve goals
- Emphasises multi-planar and functional movement focused on anatomical chains and slings
- Is designed to integrate into a range of fitness program designs and resistance training models, and
- Provides for assessment, regression, and progression with each step.

Animal Flow® includes a wide range of exercises and movement combinations that are grouped into six components, each designed to elicit specific results. These can be mixed and matched in many ways, and you can incorporate one, some, or all of them in your workouts. The six components are: wrist mobilisations, activations, form specific stretches, travelling forms, switches and transition, then the Flow itself.

Here's a quick overview of some of the components, with sample key movements:

---

46 Content here is based on material provided to FTI by Animal Flow® and is reproduced with permission.

1. ACTIVATIONS

Activations are static holds used to connect the body's system before a workout. This is an excellent movement prep exercise, while at the same time being specifically beneficial for shoulder, hips and spine (core) stabilisation.

Sample activation: Static Beast

Movement Execution

- Kneel on all fours, placing hands shoulder-width apart and knees and feet hip-width apart. The knees are slightly in front of the hips, just beneath the navel.

- Then 'Activate Your Beast': Keeping the elbows fully extended and the core active, lift the knees one inch off the ground and hold.

Sets and reps: These are performed as timed sets. The set stops as soon as you can no longer maintain form. An example would be working up to 2 minutes, using 30-second sets.

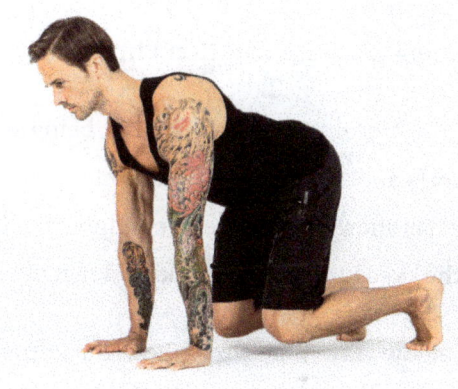

2. FORM SPECIFIC STRETCHES

Form specific stretches are full body stretches that start in an animal form and then move through various ranges of motion. The goal is to encourage full body mobility and stability. We explore opposing end ranges, like flexion followed by extension or internal rotation followed by external rotation. These stretches should be performed with control. The end points can be held for greater time in order to make the stretch static or moved in and out of as an active/dynamic stretch. These are great for correcting postural distortions and balancing the joints.

Sample form specific stretch: Crab Reach

Movement Execution

- Begin in a crab position by placing the hands slightly wider than shoulder width. The fingers should be pointing the opposite direction from the toes. This places the arm in external rotation, which opens up the front of the shoulder joint.

- There should be roughly equal distance from hips to hands and hips to heels, one inch off the ground.

- Bring the reaching arm up, about 20 cm from the face.

- Start pushing the hips up toward the ceiling, being sure to push through the heels and squeeze the glutes. Once you can get into a full '3 Point Bridge' (as shown in picture 2), continue to follow the hand around with the eyes until you are looking down toward the ground.

- The reaching elbow stays bent throughout the entire movement. In the full reach position, the upper arm is completely relaxed, framing the head.

Reps and sets: This exercise should be performed as slow reps. You can hold the end position as long as you like, but for at least 3–5 seconds per rep. Perform each arm for 10–15 reps and do at least 3 sets. This exercise can also be performed as a superset or as a circuit with other exercises that use a lot of flexion at the hips, serving as an antagonistic movement.

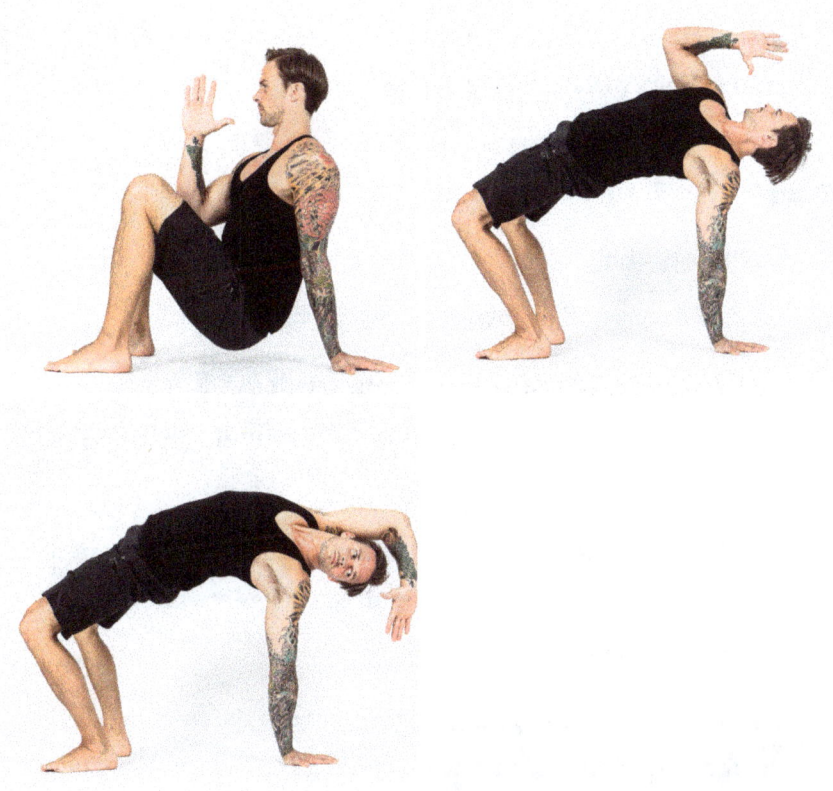

3. TRAVELLING FORMS

Travelling forms are exercises that mimic the movements of animals, allowing us to improve the function of the human animal. These versatile exercises are incredible for full body conditioning as well as warm-up and active rest. They can be used as opposing patterns to make sure that the exerciser is working in more than one plane of motion or direction. This helps create more of a balanced program and cuts down on the potential for injury that could be brought on by pattern overload.

Sample travelling form: Lateral Ape

Movement Execution

- Start in a deep squat, known as a Deep Ape.

- Reach across the body and make contact with the floor, with the back hand landing on the floor in front of the front foot (left foot if travelling left).

- Press down into the ground as you simultaneously press out of the legs. As the feet leave the ground, pull the knees toward the chest and the heels toward the hips.

- Back foot will land first, lining up directly with the front hand. The front foot will then land just before pulling hands from the ground and sinking into the next Deep Ape.

Reps and sets: These are best performed for distance rather than reps; it works well to take 10–15 metres and work one direction per set. Form is of utmost importance so be sure to stop as soon as form breaks down. If space is limited, perform one rep per direction. As you gain more balance and control, challenge yourself to hold the tuck balance longer.

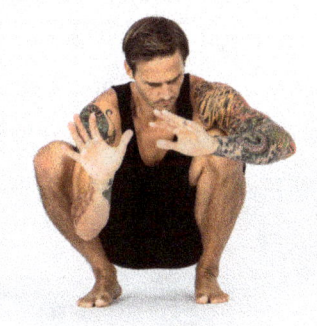
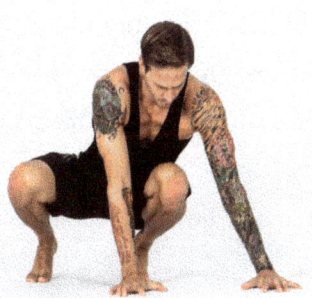

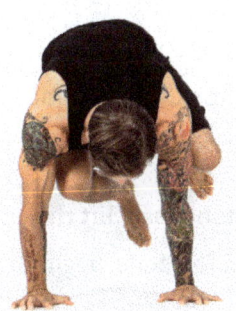
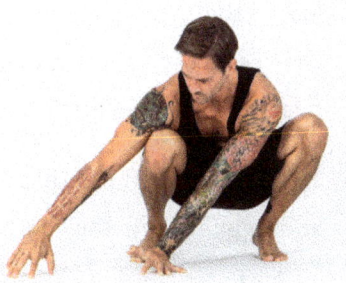

PILLAR 2: DEVELOP PROPER MOVEMENT PATTERNS

4. SWITCHES AND TRANSITIONS

Switches and transitions are dynamic movements that we perform in sequence, creating the 'flow' in Animal Flow®. They can be used to transfer from one animal form to another or to other moves within this category. There are many ways to use them within flows, although each move can also be repeated alone as a drill.

Sample switch and transition: Underswitch

Movement Execution

- Just as the name implies, the travelling leg will always be moving *underneath* the body. Begin in either the Static Crab or Static Beast position. (In the pictures we are starting in a Static Beast.)

- To perform a Left Leg Underswitch, simultaneously lift the left leg and right arm. As they both pull in toward the body, begin to rotate.

- Drop the heel in order to stop the rotation and set yourself in the crab position.

- Once stable, the travelling arm and leg can come down to connect with the ground.

Sets and reps: This movement can certainly be drilled for rotary endurance or could be randomly called out by the coach in order to work on reaction time. Perform at least 10–20 each leg per set.

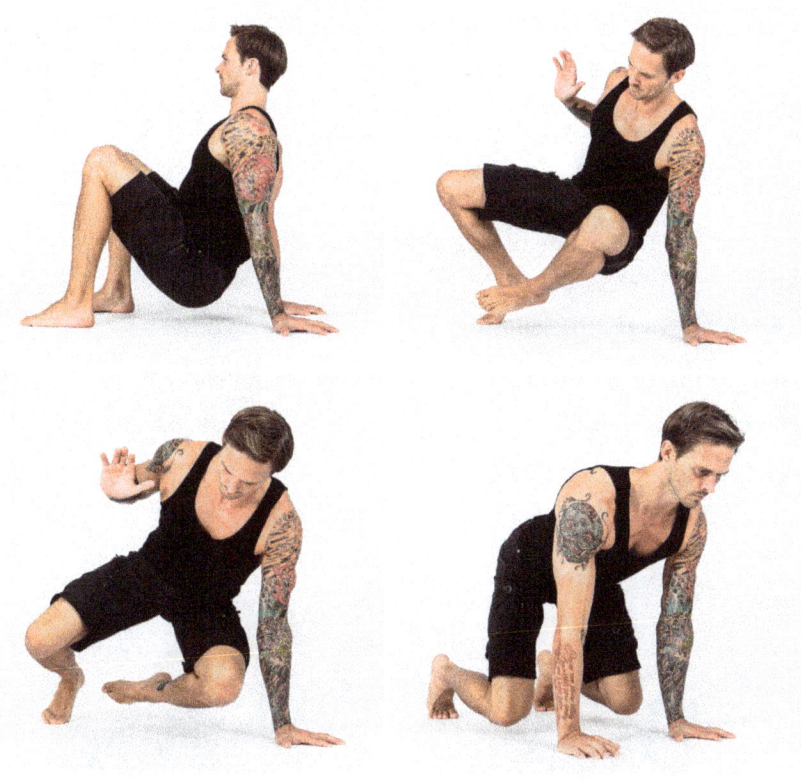

Sample switch and transition: Side Kickthrough

Movement Execution

- Begin in the Static Beast position. To perform a Right Leg Side Kickthrough, simultaneously lift the right leg and left arm.

- It's important to know that both the base foot and kicking leg should end up pointing at a 90-degree angle from the position you're starting in. The call out leg will begin to travel underneath the body (just like an Underswitch) but the eyes will now go to the rotating foot.

- As soon as the toes line up with the direction we are kicking toward, you'll drop the heel to stop the rotation. Once the heel drops, that's your green light to kick the leg.

- As the leg extends, the opposite elbow will pull the other direction. The kick leg should be extended at the knee, toes pointed and leg externally rotated from the hip.

- The elbow should be just below shoulder level and at a 90-degree angle (or less).

- Reverse the movement to get back to Static Beast.

Sets and reps: 15–20 reps can get the heart rate up quite a bit. We recommend learning the movement slowly; once it's locked in you may add speed to the equation as long as perfect form can be maintained. This is excellent for speed of rotation.

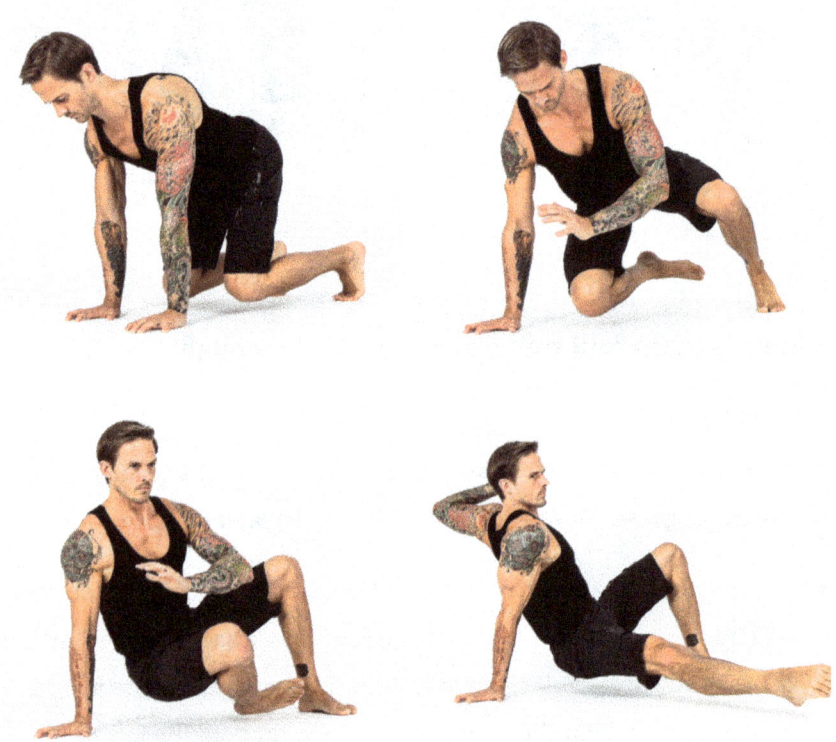

 ONLINE RESOURCE: To watch the instructional video compilation, visit – http://functionaltraininginstitute.com/book-resources/

Recap

Developing proper movement patterns is an important part of the client's journey. Our clients need to extensively cover the primal patterns to develop neuromuscular and proprioceptive awareness in movement practice. Understanding the fascial slings adds to the coach's ability to program stability in addition to the mobility we covered in Pillar 1. Two tools for achieving these aims are suspended fitness straps and crawling and ground-based work as seen in the Animal Flow® training system.

Coupling Pillars 1 and 2 into a client's program can take weeks, but when the system is followed you will see the payoff in your client's training capacity. After this phase, Pillar 3 can be effectively incorporated.

Pillar 3 – Load the Foundations

Once the foundation of our client is set, we can then begin the process of developing a progressive and functional strength program by adding external load to the equation.

One aim of Pillar 3 is to instil patience and good coaching practice into the loading phase. I have seen too many coaches who make things up on the fly and disregard the necessary steps in building incremental and progressive programs for their clients. As a coach you need to be educated about incremental loading, and you need to educate your clients in order to help them to trust and follow the path you have set out for them.

To get a clear picture of what loading the foundations looks like, we will go through a series of progressed exercises that add a layer of stability along with strength, covering several primal patterns. We cover the key strength lifts using a particular tool: the functional bag. The term 'functional bag' includes powerbags and sandbags, both of which are excellent tools for this phase of the Adaptive FTS.

Before we cover the key exercises using the functional bag, however, we take a deeper look at why loaded movements are important in training the stabilisers of the body, activating the sling systems and coordinating force transmission. We also look at why the functional bag is a versatile tool for this phase.

Training the stabilisers of the body

In Pillar 1 we learned the importance of restoring function and movement with important activation, release, stretch and mobilisation methods. In Pillar 2 we looked at how vital it is to develop proper movement patterns with good neural control and coordination in a pre-loaded state.

Now we explore why it is essential to train the stability system in order to enhance functional strength and power phases (which we will explore more in the programming section).

The landmark theoretical model of spinal stability was put forward by the pioneering researcher Manohar M Panjabi.[47] His theory led to the creation of an exercise approach to spinal stability, and more recently an adaption of this model has been applied to various other joints in the body.

According to Panjabi's theory, failure of any movement component will cause all other subsystems – whether stability or mobility, passive, active or neural – to compensate. This will result in impaired movement, regardless of the original cause.

Enter functional training. This style of training has the greatest effect on the active system. As Mark Vella describes in his book *Anatomy for Strength and Fitness Training*, 'Stabilising muscles' prime purpose is to maintain the stability and alignment of the rest of the body, so that the effective movement can be performed without unwanted bodily actions.'[48] Loading the client's foundation and challenging the active stability system increases the trainable effect on the stabilising muscles of the body.

Interestingly, not all muscles in the body are able to function as stabilisers. Some muscles exhibit a tendency to be stabilising (also known as local muscles) while others exhibit a tendency to be mobilising (global muscles). For example, in the spine, the multifidus and transverse abdominis muscles provide segmental stability to the vertebral joints, stabilising the trunk when arm or leg actions take place. In the shoulder, the rotator cuff muscles stabilise and align the shoulder joint during movements that involve the shoulder and arms.

In contrast, many of the body's larger muscles often (but not always) act as mobilising muscles, whose job it is to create movement. For example, the

---

47 Manohar M Panjabi, 'The stabilizing system of the spine. Part I. Function, dysfunction, adaption, and enhancement', *Journal of Spinal Disorders*, vol. 5 no. 4, 1992, pp.383–9.

48 Mark Vella, Anatomy for Strength and Fitness Training: An illustrated Guide to Your Muscles in Action, New York, McGraw-Hill Education, 2006, p. 23.

bicep muscle mobilises when moving the forearm toward the upper arm in bicep curls. One of the key benefits of functional fitness training is the combination of asymmetrical loads (kettlebell, sandbags and so on) with three-dimensional movement (lunges, squats and so forth). These stimulate the body's inherent stabilising systems to action, which means stimulating stabilising muscles to act as stabilisers (controlling joint position and alignment) and mobilising muscles to act as mobilisers (creating movement).

However, when we perform exercises in a one-dimensional environment, such as performing a strengthening exercise in a pin-loaded machine, the requirement for positional stabilisation is negated. Therefore, stabilising muscles are not stimulated, and the muscular system does not operate in its natural state.

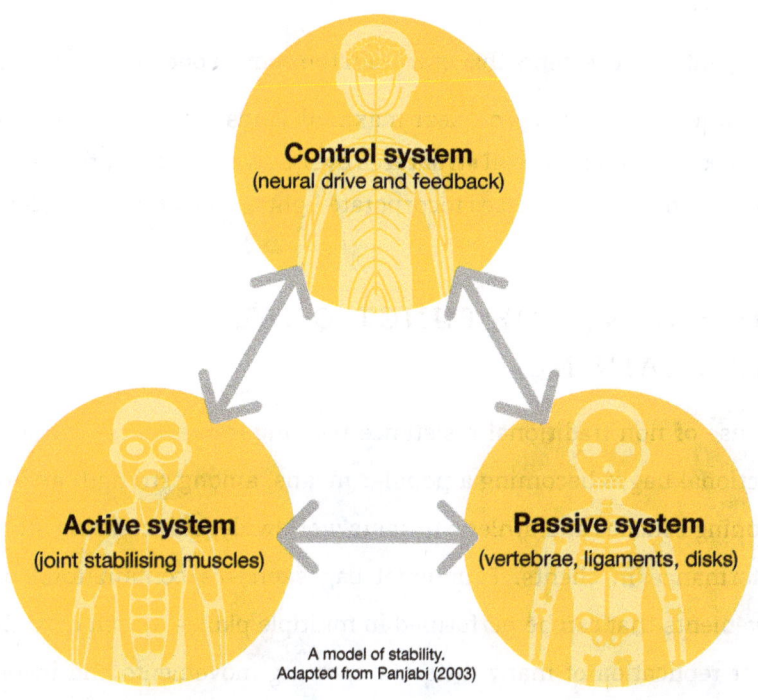

A model of stability.
Adapted from Panjabi (2003)

RECRUITING THE SLING SYSTEMS

We covered the main theory of the body's sling systems in Pillar 2; in this pillar, we need to consider how loaded movement has an effect on these systems.

Interestingly, research now suggests that the fascial slings may respond more favourably when trained with a wide variety of vectors – in angle, tempo and load.[49] It appears the fascial system as a whole responds better to variation rather than repetitive programming. To maximise the training effect on these fascial lines:[50]

- Use whole-body movements that engage all the muscles in each respective fascial line.
- Incorporate exercises that have a dynamic pre-stretch.
- Vary the lifting tempo, as training with a wide variety of lifting tempos may stimulate the strength of different fascial structures.

It is also best to avoid:

- Repetitive movements that only train the body in one movement plane.
- Training with heavy or near-maximal loads, as heavy loads may weaken different fascial structures over time. To prevent this, ensure your functional exercises incorporate light to moderate lifting loads.

THE SCIENCE OF FUNCTIONAL BAG TRAINING

The use of non-traditional resistance training implements such as the functional bag is becoming a popular means, among strength and conditioning coaches and athletic trainers worldwide, of increasing athletic performance in clients. Functional bag exercises contain total body movements that can be performed in multiple planes, which may allow closer replication of many different sporting movements and increase core muscle activation.[51]

---

49 PA Huijing, 'Epimuscular myofascial force transmission: a historical review and implications for new research', *Journal of Biomechanics*, vol. 42, 2009, pp.9–21.

50 TW Myers, *Anatomy Trains E-Book: Myofascial Meridians for Manual and Movement Therapists*, London, Elsevier, 2013.

51 PW Winwood et al., 'How coaches use strongman implements in strength and conditioning practice', *International Journal of Sports Science and Coaching*, vol. 9, no. 5, 2014, pp. 1107–25.

Therefore, an important advantage of non-traditional resistance training is the significant level of core and hip muscle engagement. Research supports this notion: in one study, researchers observed very large levels of core and hip muscle activation in response to common strongman exercises, including the farmer's walk and suitcase carry.[52] Strongman exercises such as these are well suited to the functional bag.

Non-traditional resistance training implements such as functional bags also provide the opportunity to incorporate dynamic resistances into traditional exercises such as squats, deadlifts and power cleans, rather than the constant resistance that occurs when these exercises are performed with barbell or dumbbell training. Dynamic resistance may also closely replicate the types of resistance common in many contact sports.

Taken together, these data suggest incorporating non-traditional resistance training implements and training programs may be beneficial for core and hip muscle strengthening and provide a means of specific strength training for many different contact sports.

Here are the key benefits of the functional bag that will help you to build and load your client's foundation:

- **Portability:** Functional bags are handy in group circuits as they do not require large spaces, and exercises can be easily modified without having to change weight plates.

- **Adaptability:** Functional bags can be incorporated in existing metabolic circuits, providing an alternative form of resistance training or augmenting the intensity of workouts.

- **Variety:** There are endless exercise variations possible with a functional bag, including plyometric exercises, Olympic lifting exercises, power-lifting exercises and strongman exercises.

---

52   SM McGill et al., 'Comparison of different strongman events: trunk muscle activation and lumbar spine motion, load, and stiffness', *Journal of Strength and Conditioning Research*, vol. 23, no. 4, 2009, pp. 1148–61.

- **Modification:** The functional bag allows traditional strength exercises to be performed dynamically, statically or as a combination of both. In addition, the functional bag can be used to perform both isolated and multi-joint muscle group training.

- **Stability:** Functional bag exercises effectively recruit important core and hip stabilising muscles, through the shift in load.

- **Transfer:** Functional bags allow you to create exercises that replicate both sporting and daily life movements, thus increasing the transfer of strength gains made in training to the sporting field or improving functional capacity.

- **High performance:** Functional bag exercises can easily incorporate 'velocity-based training' (VBT) principles, which can lead to increases in explosive strength, speed and power.

- **Functional:** The functional bag can be used to create multi-planar exercises, increasing the functional benefits that many traditional barbell exercises cannot safely replicate.

The exercises

1. KEY MOVEMENTS

Deadlift progressions

The hinge movement is often not used well in training sessions. At FTI we focus heavily on the hinge, both to address this lack and because it requires a system to progress clients from the ground up.

These next three progressions will enable you to execute a perfect Romanian deadlift. You can always take yourself or your client back to this progression as a method of instilling the movement pattern or addressing idiosyncrasies.

Progression 1: Performed to create stability and strength in the hips.

Movement Execution

- Maintain a stable base, supporting the knees on a functional bag
- Drill the toes into the ground and ensure heels are pointed toward the ceiling
- Hinge at 30 degrees and grip the handles in a neutral grip
- Before lifting, spread the handles apart, maintain neutral spine and drive the hips forward
- Ensure terminal extension of hips while eyes are looking toward the horizon

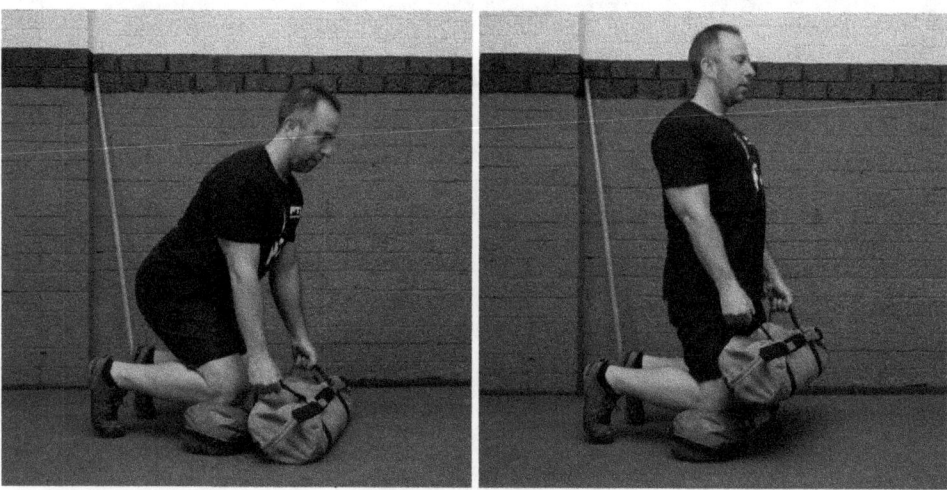

Progression 2: Performed once movement is initiated from the hips.

Movement Execution

- Have bag raised onto another bag or something of similar height, like a Reebok step
- Plant the feet into the ground and initiate a hinge movement
- Using a neutral grip, spread the handles apart, maintain neutral spine and drive the hips forward
- Finish with terminal extension of the hips and looking toward the horizon

Note: As you perform the movement, recall the functional backlines and the entire connection from head to heel. With that in mind as you lift the bag, pull using the posterior chain and the scapula.

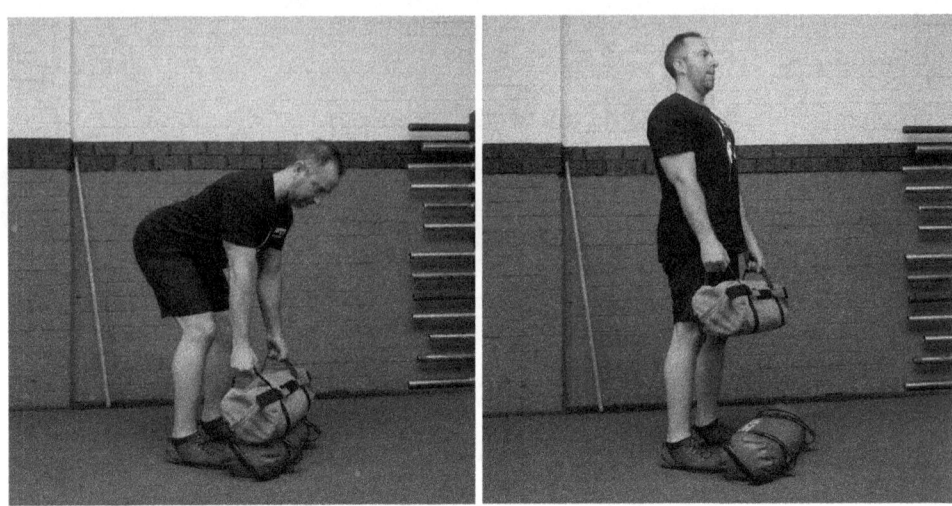

Progression 3: Performed only when range of motion is achieved.

Movement Execution

- This is the same as progression 2, except you are now lifting the bag with an increased range of motion, which makes the movement more difficult.

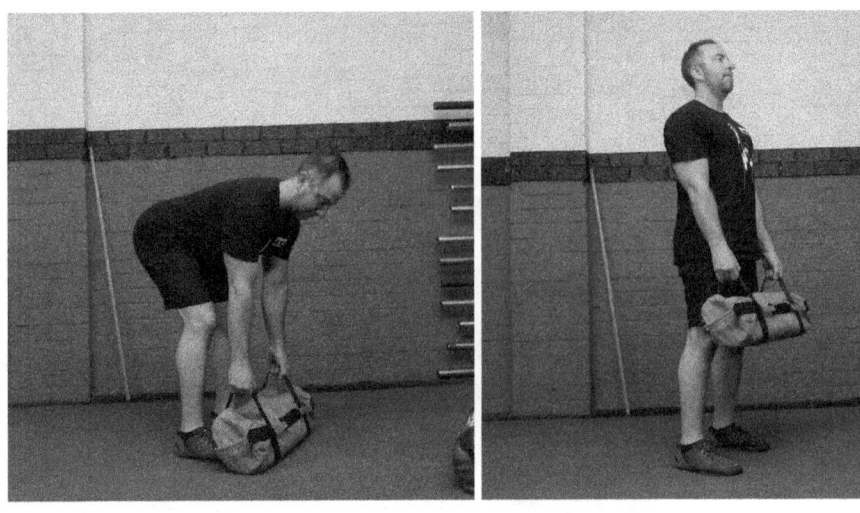

2. Standing bent over (SBO) row

This simple yet effective exercise comes in at number two because it strengthens the back muscles while maintaining a hinge position. We therefore have isometric loading of the lower back and hips; our feet are connected strongly to the ground for increased stability and neural drive. It is from the strengthening of the upper back muscles that we establish the foundation and transition into the power movement of the clean.

Movement Execution

- Have bag placed with handles in neutral position
- Come into a hinge and grip the handles
- From a stable position, pull the bag toward the belly

Note: Perform the movement with a controlled and smooth emphasis, slow on the way up (concentric phase) and slow on the way down (eccentric phase).

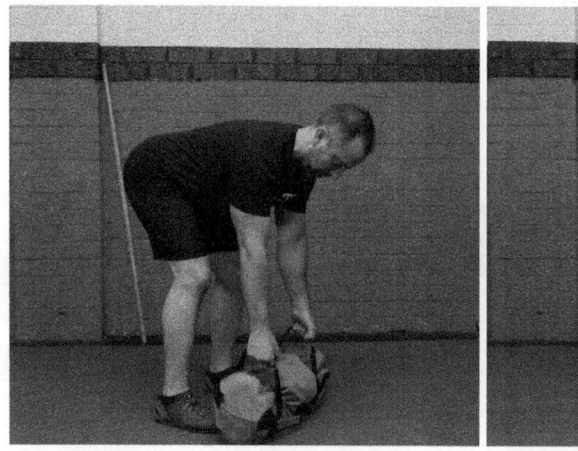
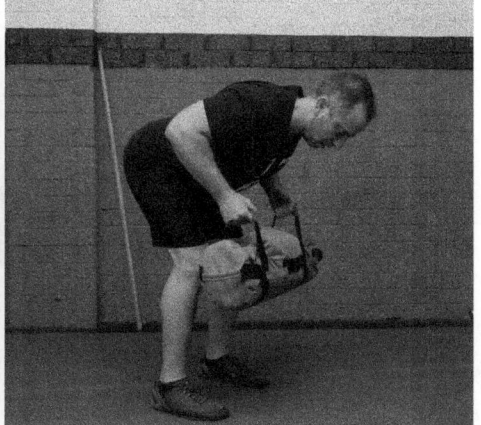

3. Cleans

The clean is a whole-body power movement that uses the ground force reaction from the feet and up the kinetic chain in one explosive and swift movement.

It is a foundational functional bag movement because it allows us to safely and effectively get the bag into the rack position, from which we perform a whole host of other strength and stability movements.

Movement Execution

- Assume a hinge position and grip the bag in neutral grip
- Explosively pull the bag from the ground in a vertical line
- Insert the hands quickly into the handles and tuck the bag into chest level
- Once in rack position, draw the elbows in and up
- Ensure your vision is not blocked by having the bag lifted too high

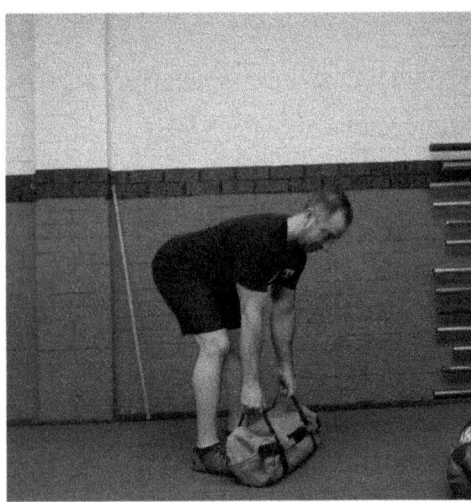
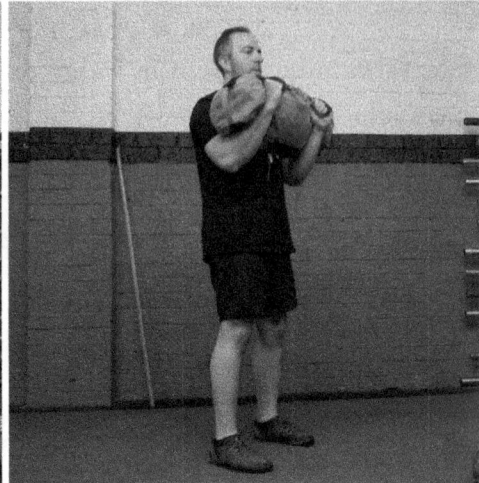

4. Front loaded squat

Arguably, front squats are the 'bee's knees' when it comes to teaching clients how to squat. This is due to the load being in front of the body, which fires the anterior sling system, thereby keeping it upright. The anterior core is engaged and working hard, as are the anterior shoulders. The more upright trunk requires greater recruitment of the quadriceps, which is beneficial for strengthening and keeping the knees aligned during movements such as walking or running.

Movement Execution

- Ensure the bag is 'hugged' into rack position with elbows raised in and slightly up
- Spread the ground away before descending into the squat
- Keep trunk upright and eyes looking toward the horizon

Note: As with the bent over row, perform the movement in a more controlled and smooth fashion: slow on the way up (concentric) and slow on the way down (eccentric).

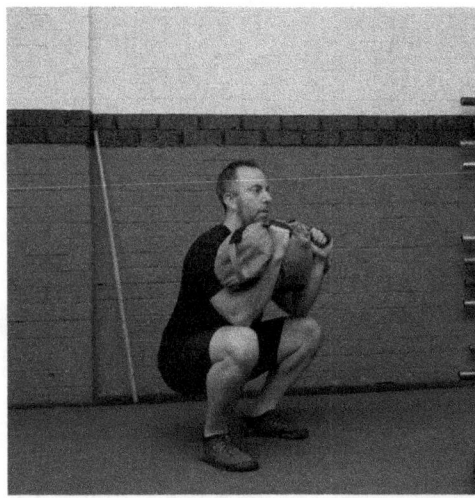 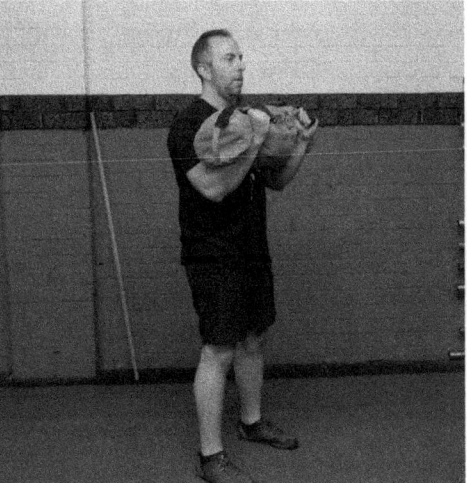

5. Lunge

The lunge, like the squat, is a fundamental movement pattern that requires good mobility in the ankles (ankle dorsiflexion). By focusing on a heel drive during push off, we can cue the client to avoid driving onto the toes instead. In addition, the activation of the posterior chain will mean we can stabilise better during concentric and eccentric loading phases.

Different lunges have different training effects. A reverse lunge is a decelerated movement, whereas a forward lunge is an accelerative movement.

Movement Execution

- Keep the bag hugged toward chest

- Keep the foot you are driving off from stable. If it is a reverse lunge, press strongly down with the left foot (as in picture 3). In a forward lunge, there is greater balance required when planting the front foot

- Keep an upright trunk as you perform the movement

- Keep eyes looking toward the horizon

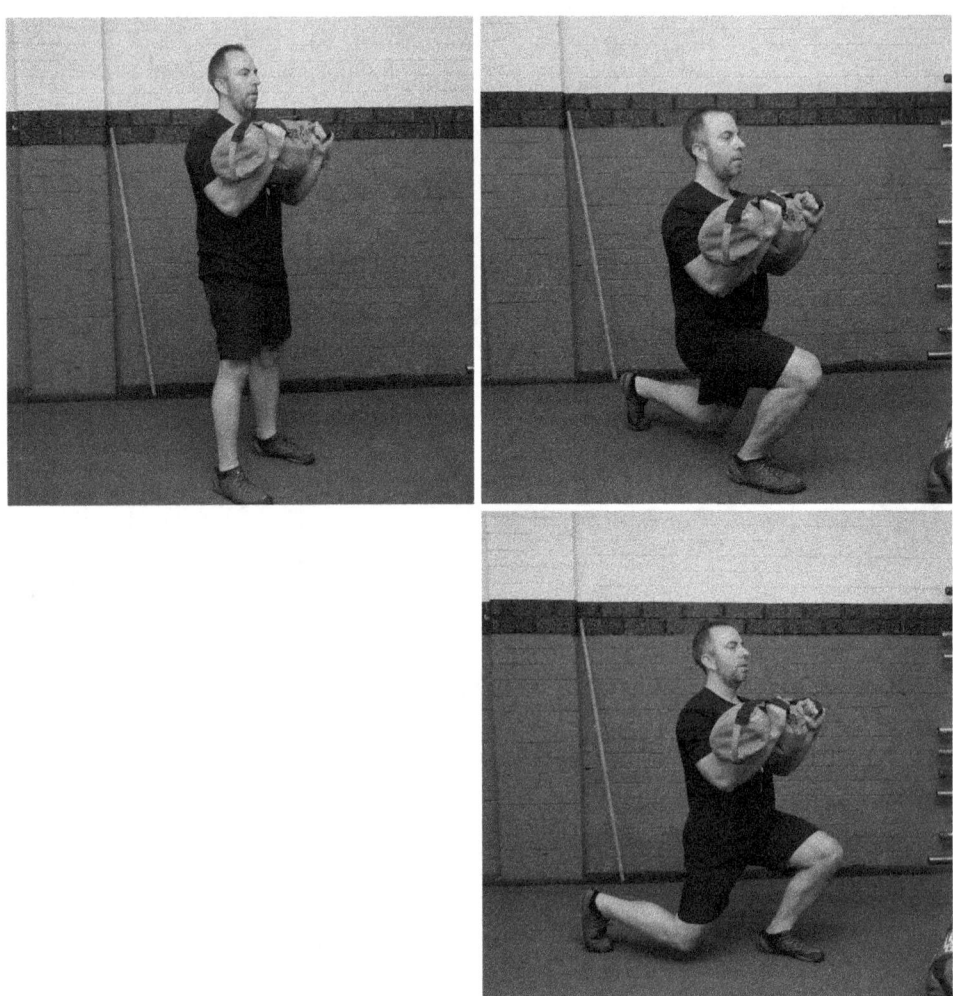

6. Press

The standing vertical press is the mother of all strength exercises. Not only are we establishing strength of the upper body, we are also learning to stabilise the core and pelvis during the movement. The neural requirements of the movement are greater than if you performed a seated press, say with a machine weight.

Vital to the movement are both slow concentric and eccentric phases of the lift. All too often it is easy to do a good lift that is controlled and smooth on the way up, only to let gravity drop the bag into rack position. It is the eccentric phase where tendon, ligament and fascial strength are trained.

Movement Execution

- As you press, keep elbows pointed forward
- Ensure the wrists remain neutral (as in picture 2)
- In finished position, keep elbows locked and hold in that position for at least one full second

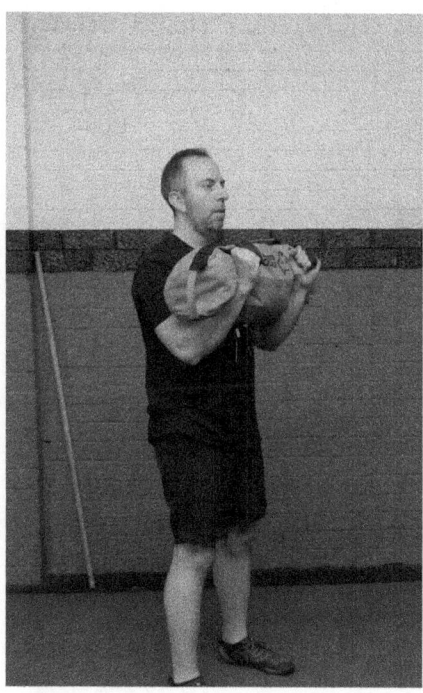
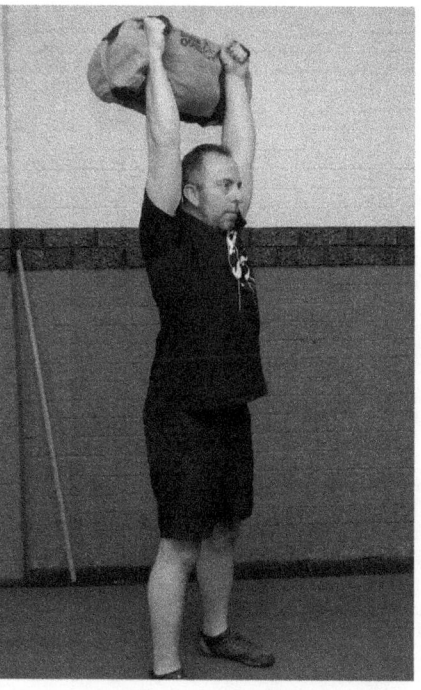

KEY LOADED POSITIONS

By simply holding the following positions under time (time under tension) we are creating necessary stability within the local stability system of the body.

Note: it is important to establish the client's baseline strength with the bag before loading them. Bear in mind that the bag needs to be heavy enough to challenge the stability system.

1. Front load

Movement Execution

- As you hold the bag, keep the knees soft and release the tension in the upper traps, which will create quicker levels of fatigue
- Breathe throughout the hold

Note: A good start is to do multiple sets for time. For example, 3 sets of 30 second holds each set.

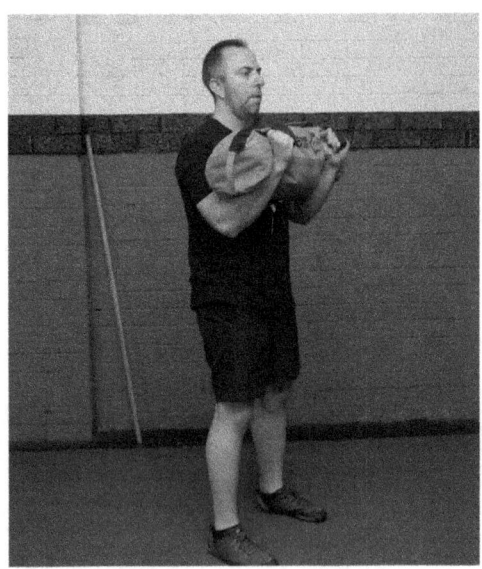

2. Overhead load

Movement Execution

- Keep full lock-out with wrists in neutral position
- Check loaded movement with bag directly above the heels and ensuring neutral spine

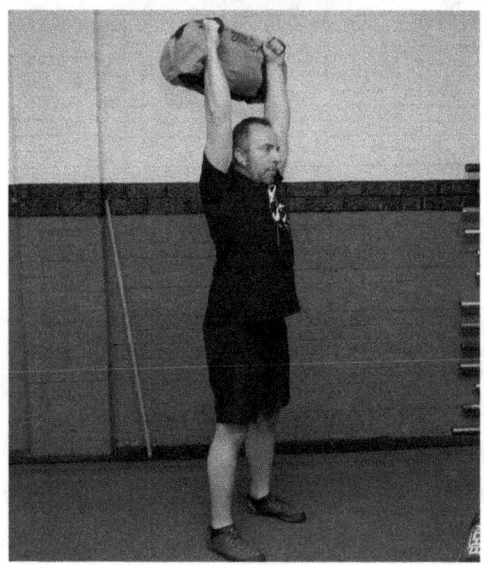

3. Shoulder hold

Movement Execution

- Keep a firm, open-handed grip on the bag
- Ensure the bag is centred on the side of the shoulder

Note: This will challenge asymmetrical stability, which is a greater challenge for beginner level clients. The lateral stabilisers will also be activated and further challenged in this particular hold.

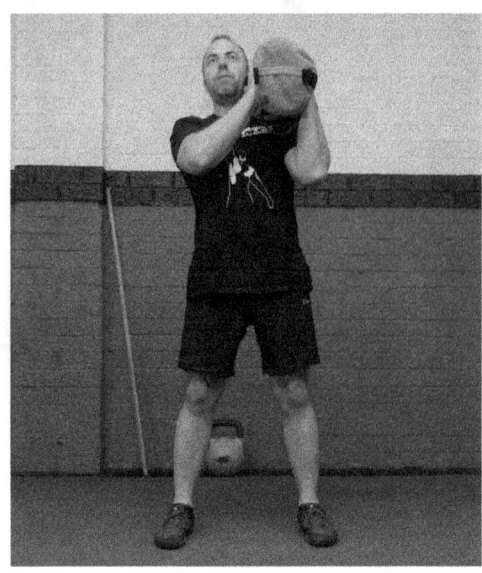

ASYMMETRICAL LIFTS

Once we have established the foundation via the key movements and loaded positions, we can begin to challenge the nervous system by creating a unilateral or asymmetrical lifting option. These are staggered stance movements.

1. Romanian deadlift (RDL)

Movement Execution

- Assume a split stance position, hinge, then hold the handles in neutral grip
- As you lift the bag, push strongly off the front foot
- Drive the hips forward

Note: The back leg is simply to stabilise. Keep the ball of the foot drilled into the ground throughout the movement.

Sling system: Longitudinal on working side and anterior and posterior throughout the movement.

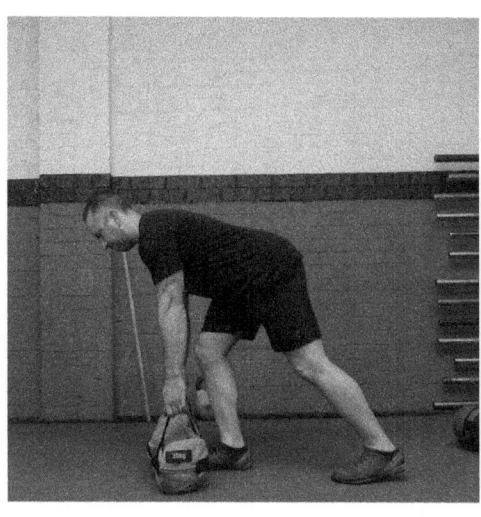
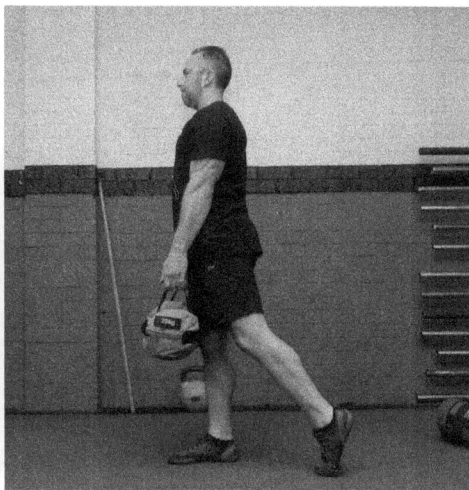

2. Bent over row

Movement Execution

- Assume the split stance position, keeping a neutral spine and neutral grip
- The key is to remain stable in the hips as you perform the row
- Notice what is happening in the hips as you begin the movement. The front foot is working more strongly to stabilise the trunk

Sling system: Anterior and posterior sling system.

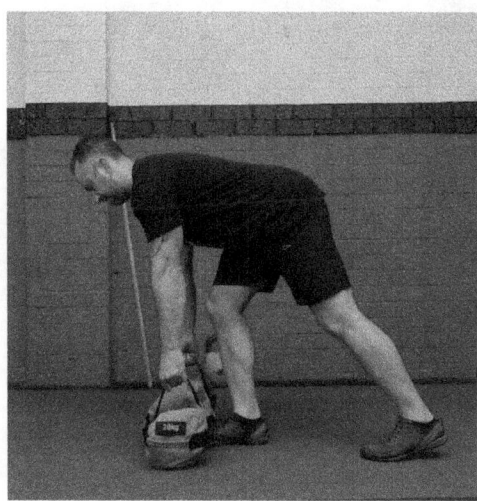
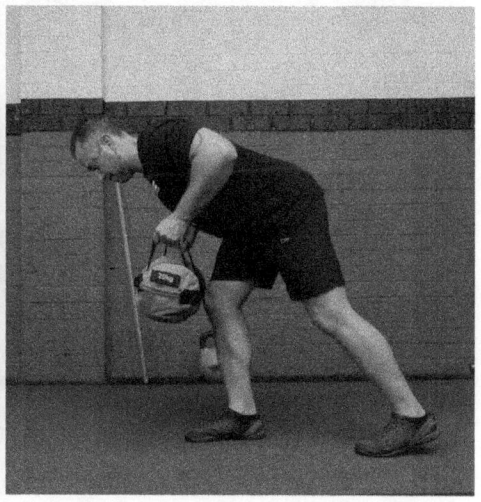

3. Unilateral RDL

Movement Execution

- This is a progression from the split stance deadlift
- You will be fighting hard to keep the hips neutral and even as you perform the movement
- The key is to work slowly throughout the movement, keeping the trunk tall, or as Nick Winkleman says, 'Head to heel, strong as steel'

Note: A useful cue is to keep the heel of the 'floating' leg pointed up, then instruct your client to gradually kick the leg out and be active with it. This will help stabilise the trunk and activate the sling system.

Sling system: Longitudinal sling system.

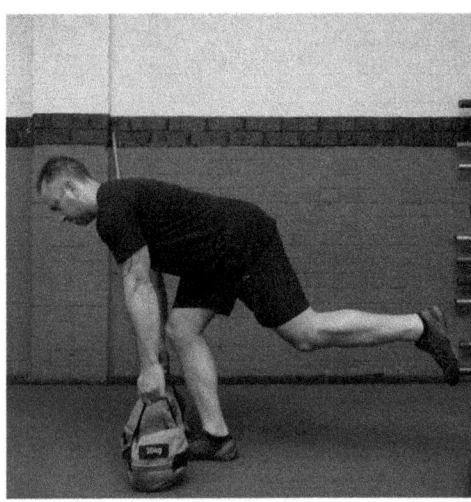 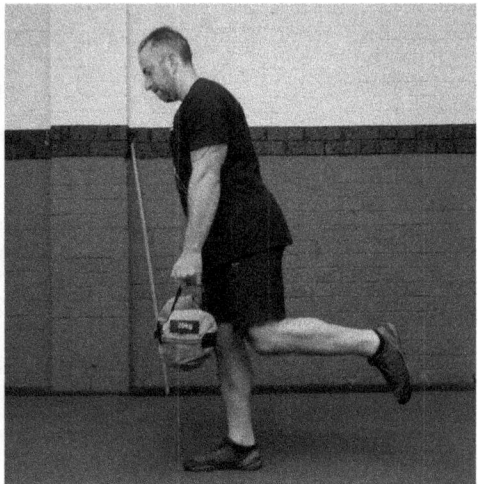

WALKS AND CARRIES

Include carries and walks in your programming if you want to build a foundation of stability and strength that is truly functional.

We first begin with a functional bag due to the soft construction of the tool. This is easier and less intimidating for clients to perform with than a hard tool. However, we still need to load our clients safely and provide a gradual increase of time under tension while performing any kind of carry. For example, we suggest beginning with multiple sets of twenty seconds under a light load rather than opting for a heavy load where the client is compensating in order to maintain hold of the object.

1. Front loaded walk

Front loaded walks are great to challenge the anterior core and shoulder strength.

Movement Execution

- Perform with small and slow steps
- Keep eyes looking to the horizon
- Keep bag hugged to chest
- Maintain constant breathing cycles as you walk by syncing your breath to each step: breathe in one step and breathe out the next step

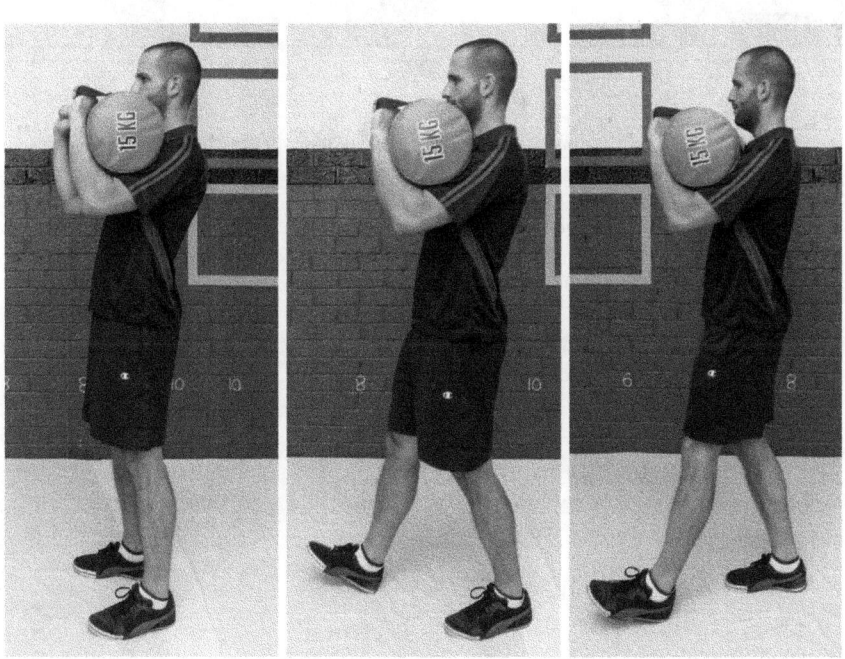

2. Overhead hold walk

Overhead walks are great for shoulder stability. This exercise challenges the posterior chain to help stabilise the trunk during each swing phase of the gait/walk.

Movement Execution

- Perform walk with small and slow steps
- Keep pressing the bag skyward
- Keep eyes looking to the horizon
- Maintain constant breathing cycles as you walk by syncing your breath to each step: breathe in one step and breathe out the next step

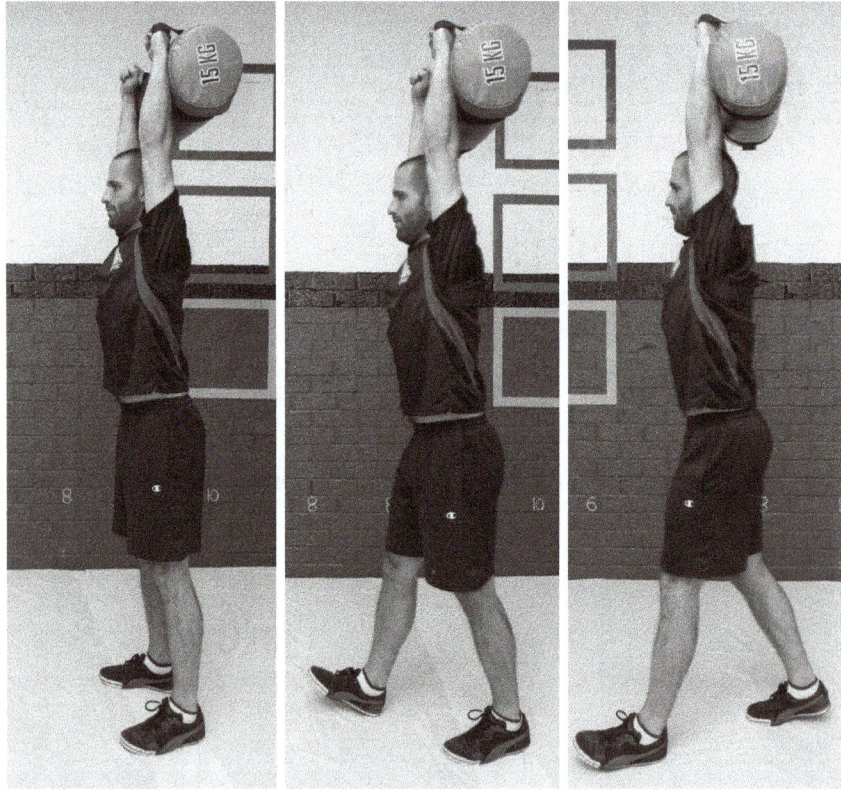

 ONLINE RESOURCE: To watch the instructional video compilation, visit – http://functionaltraininginstitute.com/book-resources/

Recap

Loaded movement is all about building a foundation of stability and strength. By introducing the hinge found in the deadlift, we are building greater levels of stability within the hip complex, particularly by recruiting the sling system. Once we begin moving efficiently from this hinge movement, we can introduce more power-based elements into our training like the swing, high pull and snatch.

The wonderful benefit of the functional bag is that it provides a seamless transition into more advanced and complex power-based training methods like the kettlebell and barbell. Having provided the foundation for these advanced movements in Pillar 3, we can now move on to exploring them in Pillar 4.

Pillar 4 – Build Strength and Power

The kettlebell is the tool of choice for Pillar 4 because of its versatility. We can train the stability system very efficiently with this non-traditional tool due to its compactness and variation in weight.

A growing body of research suggests kettlebell training can lead to significant improvements in strength, power and rapid force production. Here's some of the evidence:

- A six-week kettlebell training program, which included 12 sets of 30 seconds maximal effort kettlebell swings alternated with 30 seconds rest, was performed twice per week on maximum (half squat 1RM) and explosive strength (vertical jump height) in a group of active younger males. The results showed significant improvements in both maximum and explosive strength of the participants. In another study, a six-week periodised kettlebell training program showed significant improvements in maximum strength (1RM squat) and explosive power (vertical jump power) in a group of recreationally active and strength trained younger males.[53]

- An investigation of the force and power profiles of a two-handed kettlebell swing reported peak and mean power during a kettlebell swing are sufficient to elicit increases in rapid force production. When applied to sports specific conditioning, the kettlebell swing can be used as an additional exercise to develop rapid force production.[54]

---

[53] JP Lake and MA Lauder, 'Kettlebell swing training improves maximal and explosive strength,' *Journal of Strength and Conditioning Research*, vol. 26, 2012, pp. 2228–33; WH Otto et al., 'Effects of weightlifting vs. kettlebell training on vertical jump, strength, and body composition', *Journal of Strength and Conditioning Research*, vol. 26, 2012, pp. 1199–202.

[54] Lake and Lauder, ibid

- A ten-week study of kettlebell training in a group of moderately trained, middle-aged males and females who trained twice weekly led to significant improvements in the 3RM bench press and 3RM clean and jerk performance. The authors concluded kettlebell training could produce a transfer of strength and power to weightlifting and powerlifting exercises.[55]

- A recent study by researchers from California State University compared the effects of a four-week kettlebell training program versus an explosive barbell deadlift training program on muscular strength and power in a group of recreational resistance trained younger males. At the completion of the four-week training program, the participants who undertook the kettlebell training demonstrated significant improvements in deadlift 1RM strength and vertical jump performance.[56]

This research confirms that kettlebell training can be considered a valid alternative to traditional strength and power training, particularly in situations where access to traditional equipment is limited.

How can we take the principles and movements learned with the functional bags and transfer them into safe and best practice with the kettlebells? What makes any strength or fitness tool useful is the system behind it coupled with the coaching ability of the teacher.

Before getting to the kettlebell exercises, let's take a deeper look at some key aspects of kettlebell training and technique.

---

[55] P Manocchia et al., (2013). 'Transference of kettlebell training to strength, power, and endurance,' *Journal of Strength and Conditioning Research*, vol. 27, 2013, pp. 477–84.

[56] MR Maulit et al., 'Effects of kettlebell swing vs. explosive deadlift training on strength and power', *International Journal of Kinesiology and Sports Science*, vol. 5, no. 1, 2017..

Training with kettlebells

Many of our daily movements are performed on one leg, or with one arm. Therefore, there is a strong argument for the use of single-limb or unilateral training, to maximise the carry-over from the gym to daily life. Single-limb exercises are also very beneficial for developing general motor patterns and range of motion.

ASSYMETRICAL/UNILATERAL LOADING

One of the most important reasons to incorporate unilateral exercises into a training program is to prevent a 'bilateral deficit'. The bilateral limb deficit is the difference between the maximal force generated by muscles when they are contracted alone and the force when generated in combination with the opposing muscles. A deficit occurs when the total unilateral force is greater than the bilateral force. Simply, we can jump higher when using two legs than with one leg, but we cannot jump twice as high with two legs compared to one leg (give this a try to find out!).

Another important reason to incorporate unilateral exercises is the asymmetrical loading effect. Training studies have observed greater core and stabiliser muscle activity occurs when performing exercises with one limb as opposed to two. For example, one set of researchers compared the trunk muscle recruitment in both single and double-handed kettlebell swings to measure differences in the two swings. The results showed higher trunk muscle activation levels in the single-handed kettlebell swing as a result of the need for more stabilisation of the core muscles for balance during the movement.[57]

Unilateral training with the kettlebells can therefore improve core and stabilising muscle strength and unilateral strength, and reduce bilateral deficits – all of which carry into everyday life.

---

57 V Anderson et al., 'Core muscle activation in one-armed and two-armed kettlebell swing', *Journal of Strength and Conditioning Research*, vol. 30, no. 5 2016, pp. 1196–204..

FORCE VECTOR TRAINING

Alongside their suitability to asymmetrical loading, kettlebells are also highly useful for training force vectors.

Force vectors refer to the direction in which the force is applied, relative to the body. Research conducted in exercises with a horizontal force vector may provide greater transfer to horizontally based movements (think long jump) and exercises with a vertical force vector may provide greater transfer to vertically based movements (think a volleyball spike).

- Functional exercises with a vertical force vector direct force from the feet toward the head. These include sandbag front squats, kettlebell rack squats, lunges, overhead presses and chin-ups.

- Functional exercises containing horizontal vector forces direct force from the back of the body to the front of the body. These include kettlebell swings, cleans, snatches, sandbag hip thrusts and Turkish get-ups.

Force vectors are important to understand when designing a program for clients. Does your client require more of a vertical force (force going up) or is horizontal force more desirable for the outcome (force going forward)? A client who wants to improve her vertical jump would benefit more from movements incorporating a vertical vector force, whereas a client wanting to improve his long jump will benefit from movements that incorporate more horizontal vector forces. As noted, a kettlebell program accommodates and incorporates different vectors.

TECHNIQUE: BREATHING AND BRACING

When training grind or strength-based movements with kettlebells, the tempo is based on the concentric and eccentric system of classic strength training. The pattern of the breath is associated with biomechanical breathing.

In a squat, the eccentric phase is lowering from standing to a squat position. We take the breath in at the end point of this position. The concentric phase is rising from the squat position to standing. We breathe out at the end point, which is at the point of a finished standing position.

Classic bodybuilding will say to breathe out during the 'relaxed phase' (eccentric) and to breathe in during the 'loaded phase' (concentric). However, the loss of tension may compromise the stability of the spine. The key word here is 'during'. Classic ergonomic and biomechanical models of lower backs during lifting demonstrate that the back muscles must continually counter the resultant torque (pressure) produced by the weight/kettlebell being lifted. As we can see in the following diagram, when the kettlebell is almost at the apex of the lift, the resultant torque on the spine is at its greatest.

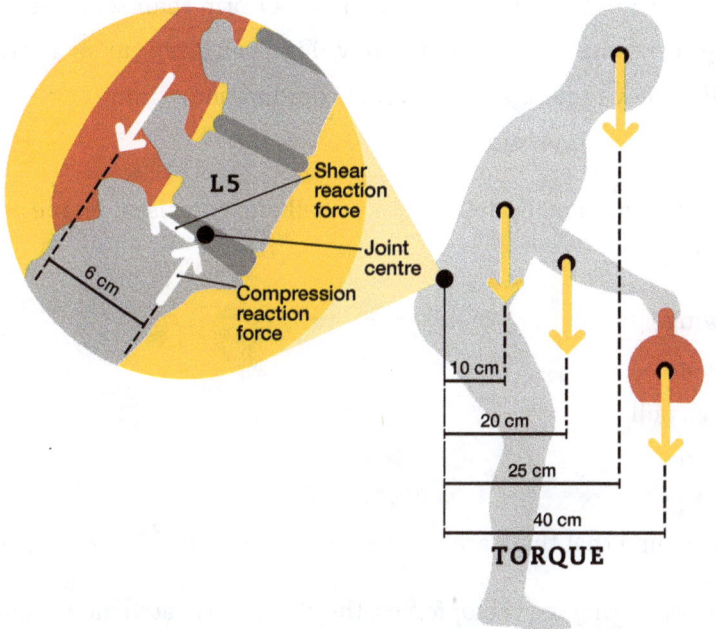

Leading biomechanical researcher Stuart McGill, in his classic textbook *Low Back Disorders,* frequently recommends bracing the core muscles during lifting tasks, as bracing will increase spinal stiffness and thus the ability to buttress the resultant torque pressures on the spine.[58] Following the biomechanical breathing technique (breathing out and pulsing a core muscle contraction at the top of the lift) when performing ballistic kettlebell exercises such as the swing, will reduce spinal pressure and prolong the health of your client's spine.

The core muscles also play an important role in maintaining adequate stability of the spine during exercise. However, these same core muscles are also required to assist our breathing as exercise becomes more difficult. This can be observed by the increased breathing rate that accompanies demanding exercise.[59] McGill therefore suggests the core muscle be trained while performing exercises that challenge breathing.

BALLISTICS

Kettlebell ballistic movements are power-based exercises that require a greater level of skill and coordination to perform than some traditional strength exercises such as a cable row, dumbbell bicep curl or a kettlebell deadlift. They require a high level of coordination, timing of movement and good use of breathing cycles.

There are traditionally four types of ballistic exercises, learned in the following order:

- Swing
- Clean
- High pull
- Snatch

Keep in mind that there are many variations of these four exercises.

For incorporating the vector forces, the clean and snatch movements can be performed with an emphasis on a vertical and horizontal vector force.

---

58   SM McGill, *Low Back Disorders*, Champaign IL, Human Kinetics, 2015.

59   JC Santana, FJ Vera-Garcia and SM McGill, S, 'A kinetic and electromyographic comparison of the standing cable press and bench press', *Journal of Strength and Conditioning Research*, vol. 21, no. 4, 2007, p. 1271.

Dead cleans and snatches employ more vertical force, while dynamic cleans and snatches require more horizontal force.

At FTI, we use a clock analogy to teach ballistics in kettlebell training.

Our model sums up the kettlebell power-based movements and provides a solid basis for understanding and teaching these movements. By understanding each 'clock hand', you will better understand the phases of each movement. You will also have a clear analogy and visual aid that can help clients move through the movement phases. When coaching the ballistic movements this model not only clarifies the phases of movement, but also highlights the horizontal vector force of the movement.

KB Ballistics clock analogy

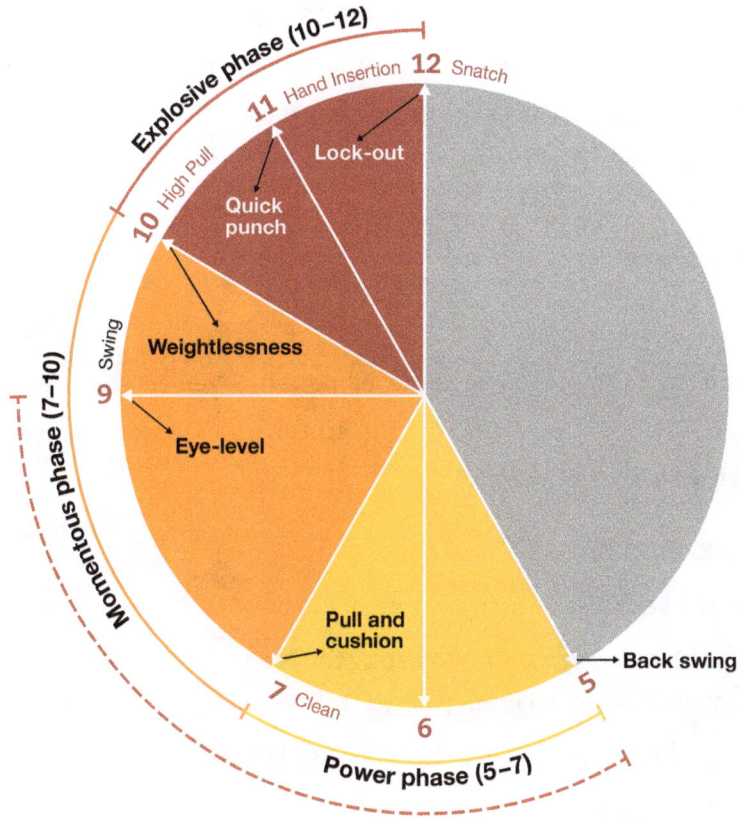

Our model sums up the kettlebell power-based movements and provides a solid basis for understanding and teaching these movements. By understanding each 'clock hand', you will better understand the phases of each movement as well as the horizontal vector force at play. You will also have a clear analogy and visual aid that can help clients move through the movement phases.

The exercises

POWER-BASED MOVEMENTS

1. Kettlebell swing

Swings, and in particular one-arm swings (OAS), help to create power via the posterior kinetic chain. In addition, the activation of the posterior sling system or superficial backline in anatomy trains, increases both the tensile and reactive strength streams of the body. Tensile strength is the rapid shortening and lengthening of the muscle, and reactive strength involves recruiting more motor neurons, which helps increase the power output during movement.

The swing is also a foundational kettlebell power movement. After first mastering the swing, in particular the one-arm swing, we move on to the clean and eventually the snatch.

Movement Execution
- Line up the kettlebell a metre in front of the body
- Reach and lengthen your back, creating the pre-tension in the posterior chain (foot to glute – picture 1)
- Pull the bell powerfully to '5 o'clock' on the clock analogy (picture 2)
- Use the free arm to counterbalance
- Snap the hips at the top phase of the movement (picture 3)

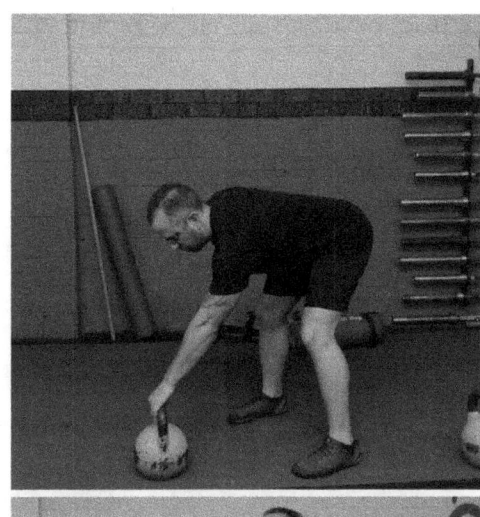
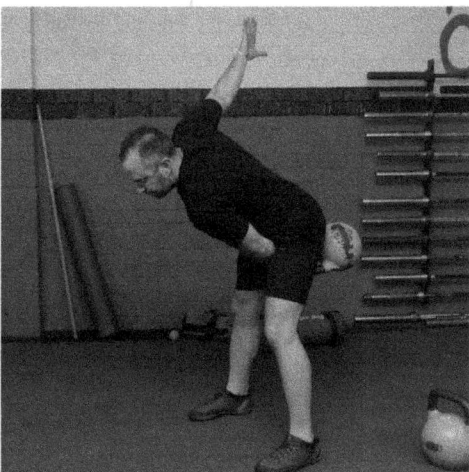
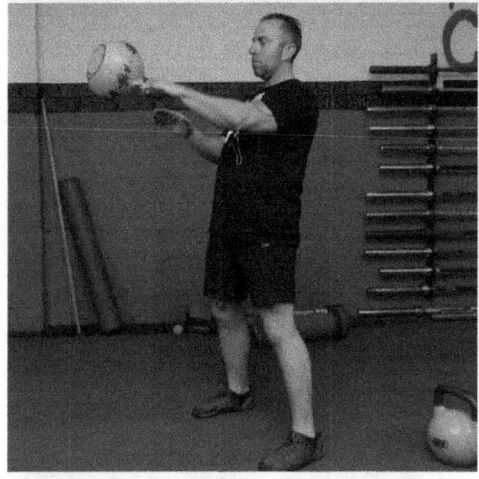

2. Clean

Kettlebell cleans use the hinge and drive element of the swing to bring the kettlebell into the fundamental rack position. Mastering the 'cushion' of the kettlebell from swing into rack (7 o'clock on the ballistics diagram) is key to this movement.

Movement Execution

- As the bell is drawn in at 5 o'clock on the diagram, employ the cue 'thumb to bum' for the internal rotation part of the movement (picture 2)
- As you drive the bell forward, 'pull and cushion' at 7 o'clock into rack position (pictures 3, 4, 5)

- To release, 'pass the dish' with palm facing up and elbow kept in to create efficiency of movement

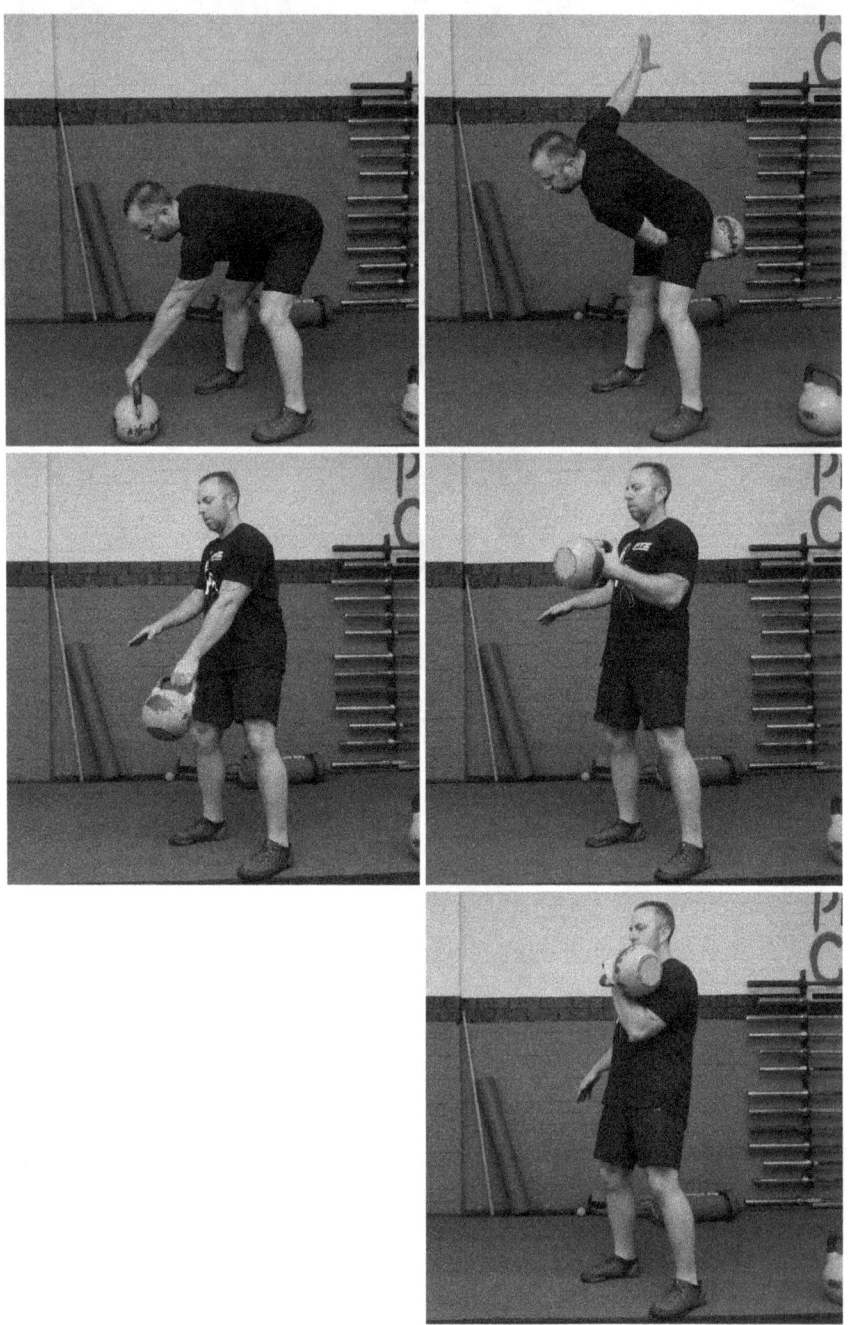

3. Snatch

The kettlebell snatch is the ultimate kettlebell power exercise. It utilises the execution elements of the swing. However, it requires greater timing and overall skill to execute. The one-arm swing brings the shoulder into a 90-degree shoulder flexion, whereas the snatch brings it to 180 degrees. A greater horizontal vector force is required to produce this movement.

Movement Execution

- To begin, bump the kettlebell forward to 6 o'clock position (picture 1)
- Back swing phase: As you hinge, thread the bell in at 5 o'clock (picture 2)
- Drive phase: Drive from the hips to 7 o'clock (picture 3)
- High-pull phase: Pull the bell in at 10 o'clock (picture 4)
- Hand insertion phase: 'Knife' the bell at 11 o'clock (picture 5)
- Lock-out phase: Finish by punching the bell to the ceiling (picture 6)

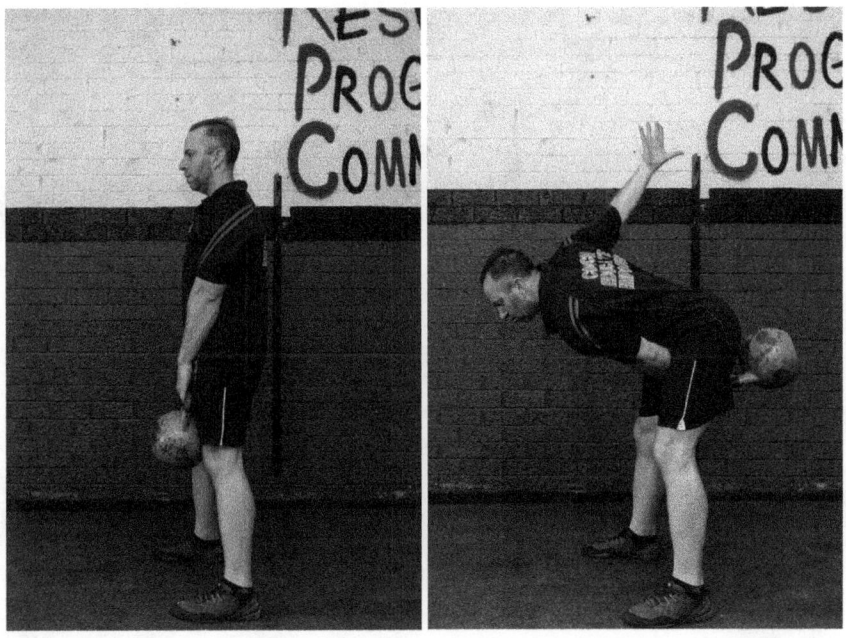

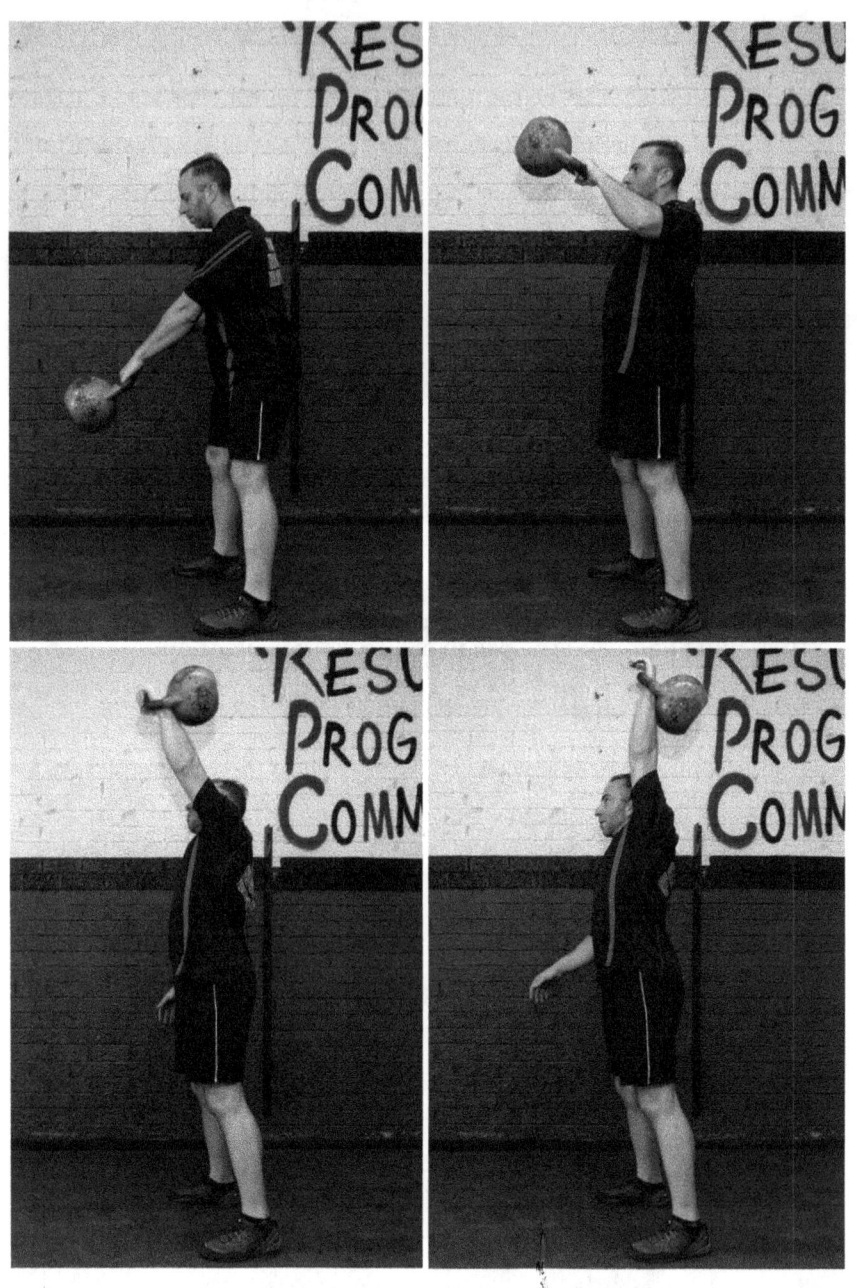

KEY STABILITY EXERCISES

Training for stability is a key component of not only kettlebell training but training functionally in general. In this section, we will look at the fundamental stability exercises using asymmetrical (or unilateral) loading. This means loading one side of the body as opposed to the weight being centred to the midline of the body, as in a goblet squat or in a more difficult barbell front squat where we have angular momentum.

1. Kettlebell (KB) rack position

The KB rack position challenges primarily:

- Anterior core
- Opposite side counterbalance (due to the asymmetrical loading)
- Anterior shoulder of the loaded side

This can be performed either as a static hold for time or as a loaded walk.

Note: Remember to perform both sides for equal time.

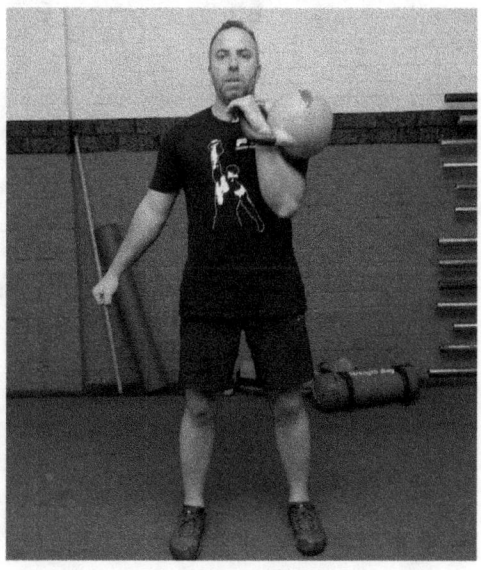

2. Overhead (OH) position

The OH position challenges:

- Shoulder stability
- Shoulder flexion
- Thoracic extension
- Core stability

This can be performed either as a static hold for time or as a loaded walk.

Note: Remember to perform both sides for equal time.

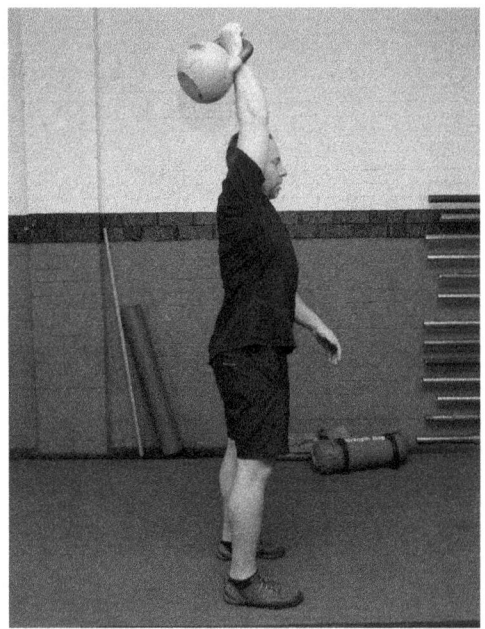

3. Single-leg (SL) Romanian deadlift (RDL)

The SL RDL challenges:

- Glute strength
- Single-leg balance
- Humero-scapular development of the loaded arm
- Posterior sling system

Note: These are best performed as repetitions and in a slow and controlled manner.

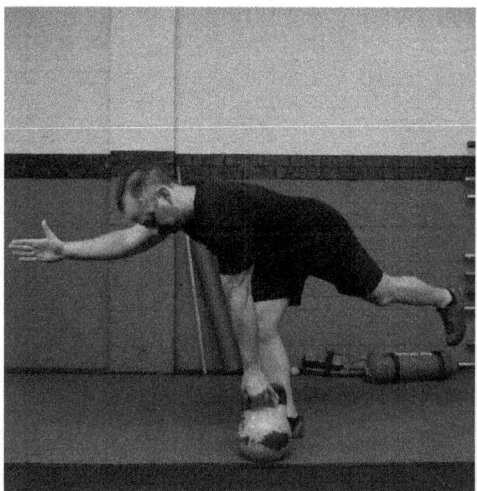
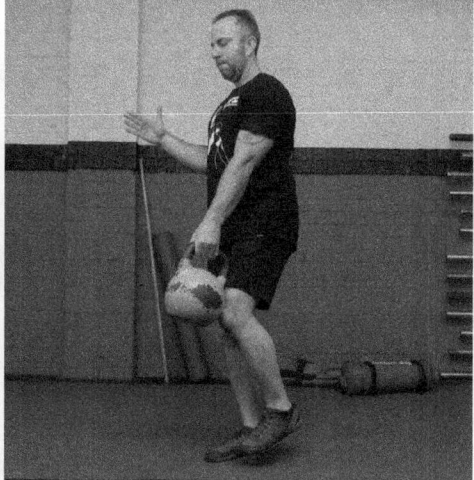

4. Lying press position

The lying chest press challenges:

- Shoulder stability in horizontal position

Note: This movement is important to practise and get right before performing the complete Turkish get-up (TGU).

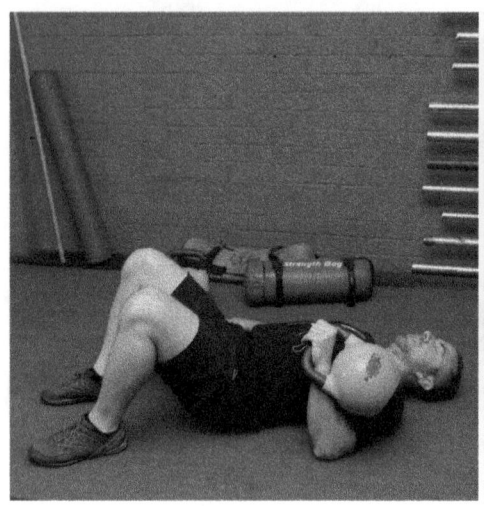
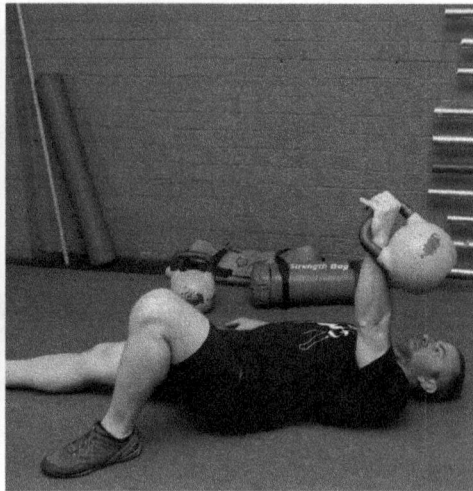

5. Bridge position of Turkish get-up

The half get-up position increases the challenge from the lying chest press for shoulder stability. In addition, it challenges:

- External obliques in the drive phase from lying position to forearm
- Hip stability and mobility in frontal plane loading

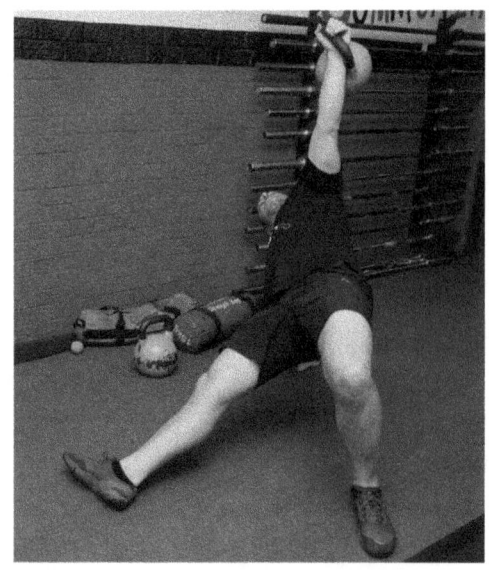

6. Bottoms-up press

The bottoms-up press here can be done as a single press, then progressed to alternating and double presses. These exercises challenge:

- Wrist stability
- Shoulder stability
- Anterior sling system

Note: This is an advanced version and should only be attempted once mastery is achieved with the previous stability exercises.

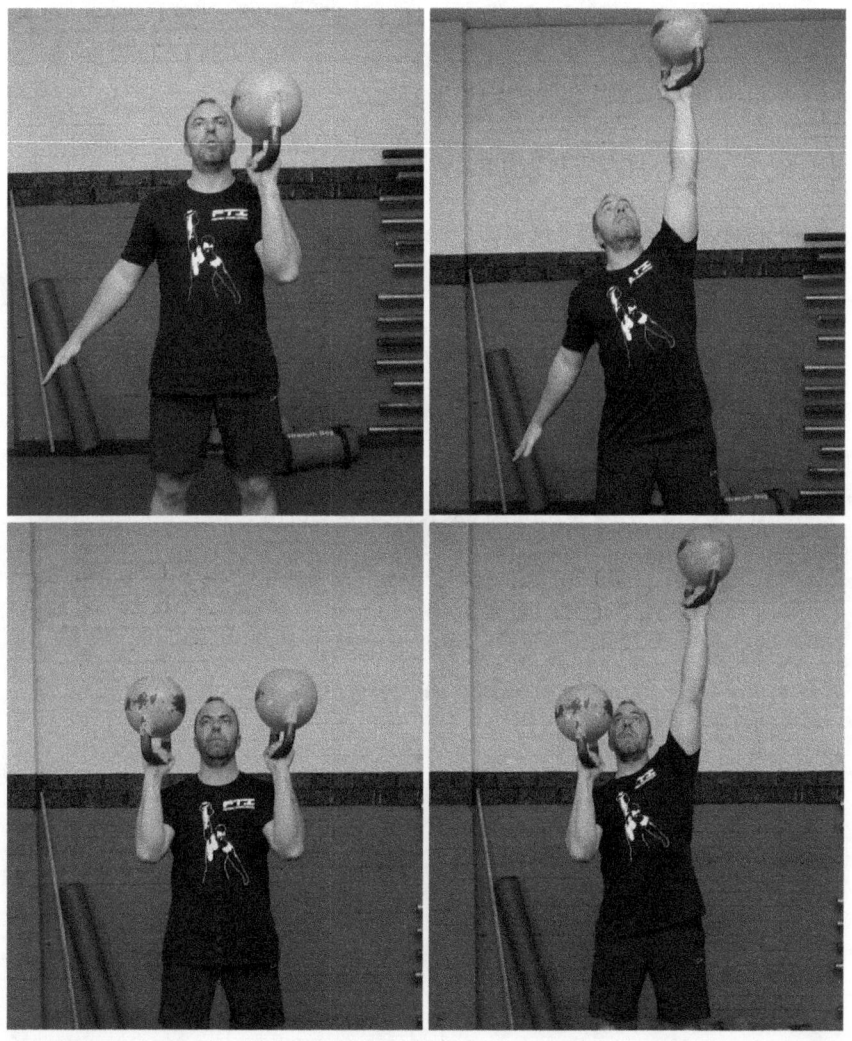

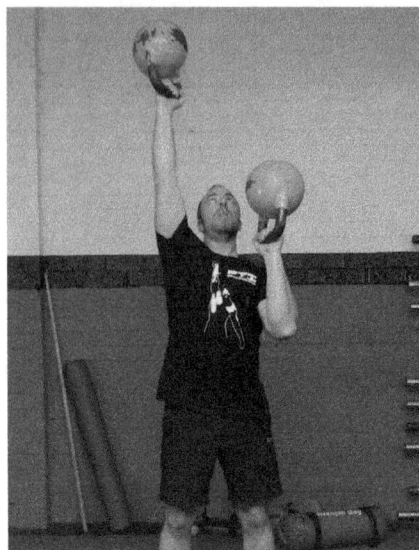 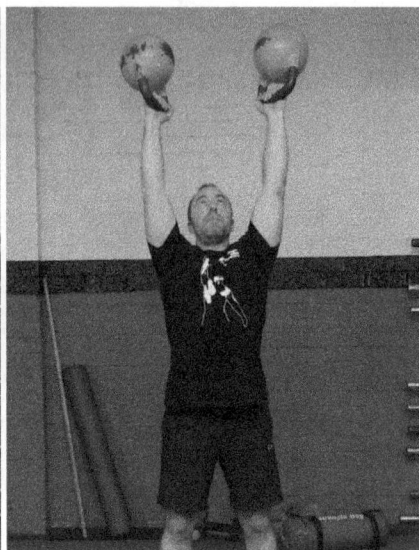

KEY STRENGTH EXERCISES

These exercises emphasise strength in relation to unilateral load, otherwise known as asymmetrical lifting.

- Strength exercises in kettlebell training are known as 'grinds'.
- These are performed with a slow tempo and clearly defined use of breath.
- With the following strength exercises, perform fewer repetitions to focus on building strength.

Note: In the power-based movements, we want to aim for a higher volume of reps if we are focusing on endurance as a training outcome.

1. Single-leg Romanian deadlift (SL RDL)

Key outcomes:

- Strengthens the glute and opposite shoulder via the posterior sling system
- Helps develop grip strength and conditioning of the forearm muscles
- Activates the free hand through the neural drive (irradiation) effect
- Helps to develop coordination and timing

Instruction points:

- Perform the movement slow on the way down (eccentric loading on the hamstrings) and slow on the way up (concentric loading on the gluteals)
- Use opposing limbs to perform the movement to target the anterior and posterior sling systems
- Avoid rotating the hips as you move through
- Keep the spine lengthened at all times

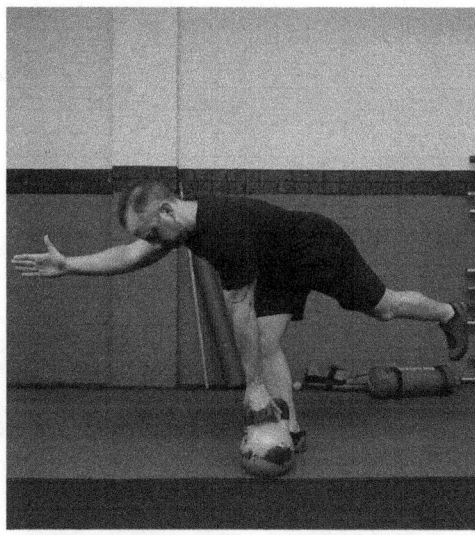 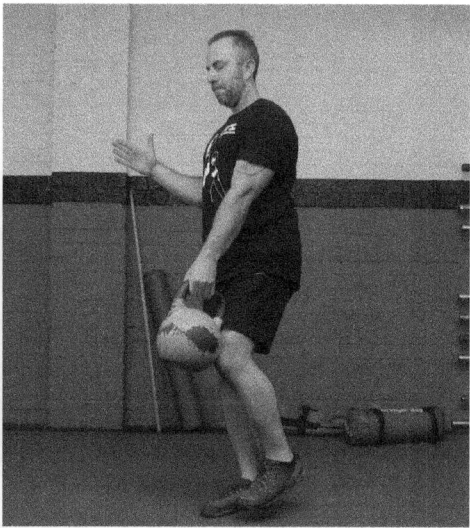

2. Kettlebell row

Key outcomes:

- Learn to create full body tension to keep the torso and pelvis neutral and balance the body during the lifting phases (eccentrc and concentric loading)
- Create strength via scapular retraction, targeting the rhomboids, lats and lower trap muscles

Instruction points:

- Ready yourself by lengthening the back limb and maintaining good alignment – 'head to heel, strong as steel' (picture 1)
- Pull the bell toward the opposing hip, ensuring the body does not rotate in the process (picture 2)
- Perform the movement slowly in the up and down phases
- Remember to breathe in at the bottom and out at the top

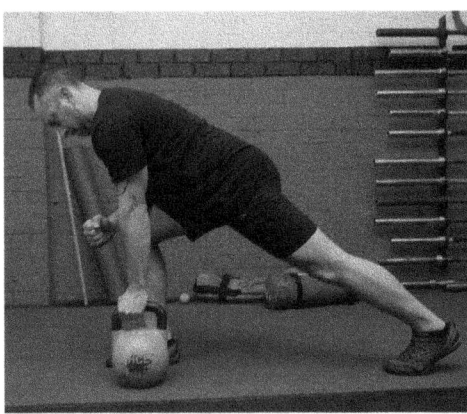
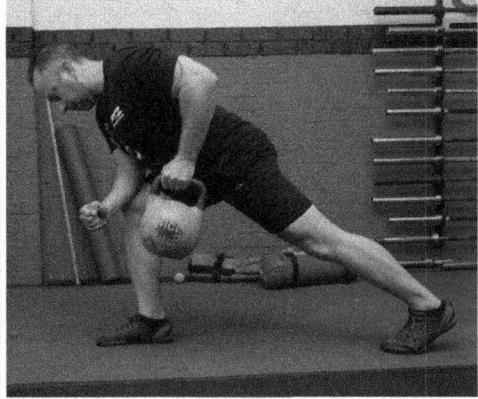

3. Kettlebell rack squat

Key outcomes:

- Create lower body strength by targeting more of the quadriceps
- Activate the unloaded side to create counterbalance
- Strengthen the anterior core
- Strengthen the anterior shoulder
- Strengthen the anterior sling system to work more efficiently

Instruction points:

- From a strong rack position (picture 1), descend slowly until you reach your depth threshold (picture 2)

Note: This threshold will differ from person to person, based on genetics and training history, particularly whether the person has been performing squats as part of a stable program.

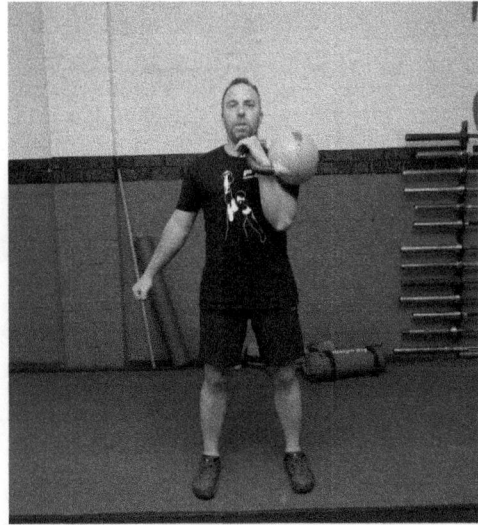
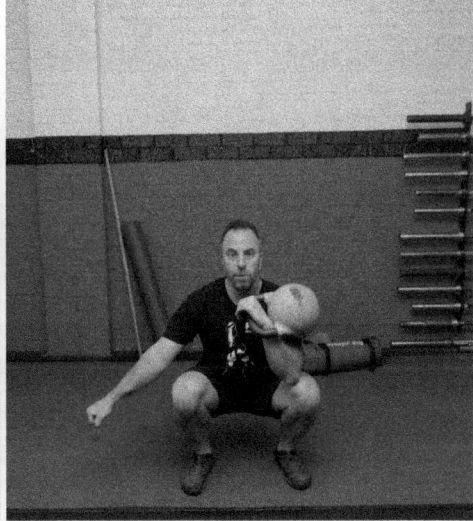

4. Kettlebell press

The kettlebell asymmetrical press is the foundational lift that prepares us to perform other challenging kettlebell movements like the Turkish get-up and the high windmill. By sustaining a strong lock-out, we also build stability into the shoulder joint.

Movement Execution

- Create neural drive by pressing feet into ground, squeezing glutes and creating tension in the free arm. (This is also known as 'Irradiating')
- Keep eyes looking forward
- As you press keep the elbow of the pressing arm pointing forward. This will keep the shoulder in a near enough neutral position.
- slowly lower the bell back into rack position and relax before creating tension again for the next repetition

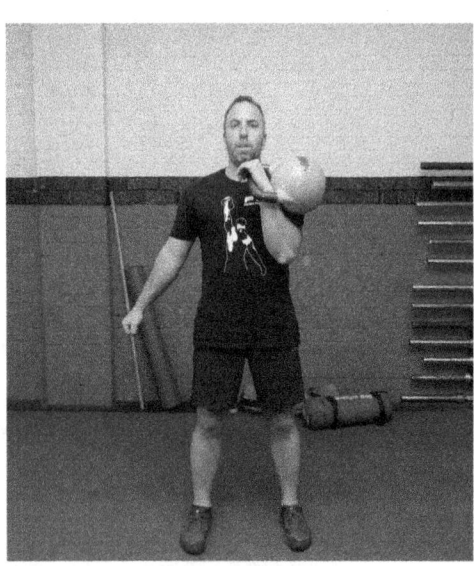
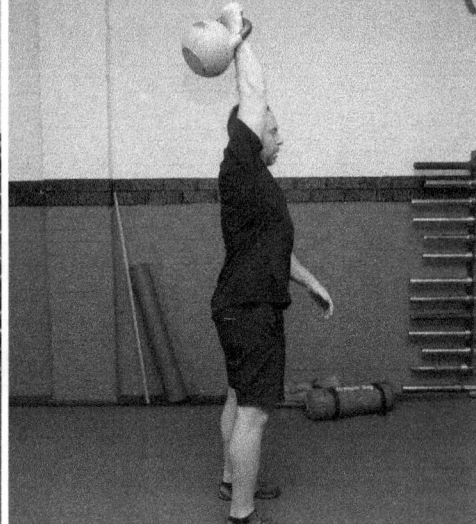

5. Kettlebell lunge

Key outcomes:

- Create lower body strength by targeting more of the quadriceps in forward lunge and glutes in reverse lunge

- Activate the unloaded side to create counterbalance – if bell is in left rack arm, step forward with right leg to load the slings. Or in a reverse lunge, step back with the left leg to activate the slings
- Strengthen the anterior core
- Strengthen the anterior shoulder
- Strengthen the anterior and posterior sling system to work more efficiently

Instruction points:

- From a strong rack position, step the leg forward or backward (depending on the goal), for example:
- If bell is in left rack arm, step forward with right leg to load the slings
- In a reverse lunge, step back with the left leg to activate the sling
- Keep the torso upright (picture 1)
- Come back to the start position smoothly

Note: Remember to reset before performing the next repetition.

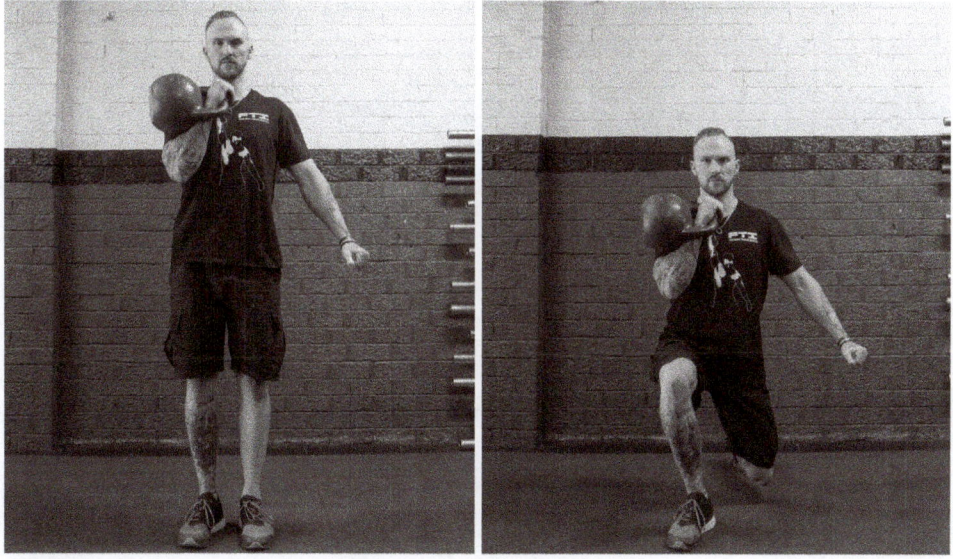

ONLINE RESOURCE: To watch the instructional video compilation, visit – http://functionaltraininginstitute.com/book-resources/

Recap

The kettlebell is a supreme training tool when it comes to building strength and power. Far from being just another strength tool, the kettlebell shows its versatility in asymmetrical loading, stability, mobility, power and endurance movements alike. The magic is in the versatility of the tool, which can be used in programming for all clients, from beginners to advanced athletes.

As we have explored, Pillar 4 is focused on building a high layer of stability, strength and power. Without being grounded in Pillar 3, which emphasises foundational stability and strength, these kettlebell exercises become a potentially dangerous method of programming because clients are simply not ready for the neural and other physiological demands of this methodology. Within the trajectory of the Adaptive FTS, however, the kettlebell exercises can produce in clients a truly functional level of strength and power. This layer of training prepares us for the complex movements of the final pillar.

Pillar 5 – Integrate Complex Movement Patterns

In the final pillar of the Adaptive FTS, we consider complex movement patterns. These are challenging movements to perform correctly, but are built on the knowledge from the previous pillars and so a logical progression from what has gone before.

Attempting a complex movement pattern is only possible once the fundamentals of the seven primary movement patterns have been performed with proficiency and within a sufficiently challenging program. Your client may perform a lunge, squat and press technically well, but can they maintain that technique when you program those movements into a workout? Integrating complex movement patterns requires both the skill to perform a given movement *and* the capacity to perform it multiple times. The skill needs to match the fitness level sufficient for a given workout.

In Part 1, *Coach with Purpose*, we discussed the importance of mastery as a way to foster motivation for clients. Motivation is found not only in goals to get fitter, stronger and more mobile, but also in the ability to develop new skills. We call this skill acquisition. Without progression and variety of movement, clients will get bored quickly. The body and mind will adjust to the neural demands of the movement. Adding complex movement patterns is a great way to provide physical and mental stimulus for the client. Mastering such patterns becomes a motivating factor in its own right, quite apart from all the fitness benefits the training of these complexes will produce. However, we need to ensure that the challenge matches the client's ability, especially when high-intensity programs are prescribed.

A large portion of Pillar 5 focuses on the battling rope as a tool, and we will therefore take a look at some of the benefits of rope work before embarking on the exercises. However, complex movement patterns can draw on all of the tools from the previous pillars; you'll find a number of other complexes in the second half of the pillar.

The battling rope

The battling rope, or 'rope' for short, is an efficient training system for targeting both the aerobic and anaerobic system. Additionally, it's a great tool for the development of power.

The rope tool has seen a dramatic rise in popularity in the fitness industry over the last few years. Historically, battling ropes have been used to achieve a variety of different physical performance goals, such as improving group cohesion during military training, improving upper body strength in high school sports programs and increasing upper body strength during gymnastics training.[60] However, in the fitness industry, battling ropes are most often used during circuit training.

But what particular benefits do battling ropes provide in a training setting? Until recently, the effect of battling rope training was unknown. However, a growing body of research now suggests training with battling ropes may provide a sufficient level of cardiorespiratory stimulus to improve aerobic fitness.[61]

For example, one study compared the metabolic demands of three different exercise sessions:

---

60 NA Ratamess et al., 'Comparison of the acute metabolic responses to traditional resistance, bodyweight, and battling rope exercises', *Journal of Strength and Conditioning Research*, vol. 29, no. 1, 2015, pp. 47–57.

61 CJ Fountaine and BJ Schmidt, 'Metabolic cost of rope training', *Journal of Strength and Conditioning Research*, vol. 29, no. 4, 2015, pp. 889–93.

- Battling ropes training: 3 sets x 30-second intervals, with each set divided into three 10-second bouts of single-arm alternating waves, double-arm waves with a half squat and double-arm slams with a half squat.

- Bodyweight circuit training: push-ups (3 sets of 20 reps with a BOSU ball, then lateral crawls for 3 sets of 10 reps with a 2-minute rest), burpees (3 sets of 10 reps with a 2-minute rest) and planks (3 sets of 20 seconds with a 2-minute rest).

- Traditional weight training: 3 sets of 10 reps at 75% 1RM of bench presses, squats, curls, bent over rows, high pulls, lunges and deadlifts.

At the completion of this study, the researchers observed the highest caloric expenditure and cardiovascular responses from the battling rope protocol.[62] A further study reached similar conclusions, finding that training with battling ropes can meet established thresholds (ACSM), known to increase cardiorespiratory fitness.[63]

Taken together, this growing body of research suggests battling ropes may be used as a modality for improving cardiovascular fitness and metabolic conditioning.

Alongside these benefits, emerging research suggests training with battling ropes can stimulate the core muscles and improve grip strength. For instance, one study examined the effects of a five-week high-intensity (20 minutes, alternating exercises every 2 minutes) battling rope training program on grip strength and body composition. At the completion of the study, the researchers observed significant improvements in grip strength.[64] In another battling rope study, the researchers investigated

---

62 Ratamess et al., ibid.
63 Fountaine and Schmidt, ibid.
64 J Meier, J Quednow and T Sedlak, 'The effects of high intensity interval-based kettlebells and battle rope training on grip strength and body composition', *International Journal of Exercise Science*, vol. 8, no. 2, 2015, pp. 1199–202.

the effect of bilateral and unilateral alternating waves on trunk muscle activity and reported that both single and double-handed waves stimulate the external obliques and spinal erector muscles.[65] These studies suggest therefore that battling rope complexes can be used to strengthen the grip and to increase core strength.

For practical application in coaching, battling ropes can:

- Impose significant cardiovascular and metabolic demands, improving cardiovascular fitness and metabolic conditioning.

- Burn up to ten calories per minute. This is comparable to traditional aerobic exercises such as running, cycling and swimming, which range from six to nine calories per minute.

- Strengthen the grip, which may have significant benefits for sports or activities that require a firm grip.

- Improve core strength. Single-arm battling rope waves impose a significant demand on the oblique muscles, while double-handed waves impose a significant demand on the spinal extensors, making both exercises a suitable choice for core strengthening.

Not only is the rope a useful tool to elicit the training effects mentioned, but it can be used as both an indoor and outdoor training tool, making it a versatile coaching choice.

---

[65] J Calatayud et al., 'Muscle activity during unilateral vs. bilateral battle rope training', Journal of Strength and Conditioning Research, vol. 29, no. 10, 2012, pp. 2854–9.

VELOCITY TRAINING WITH THE ROPE

The changing vector forces that occur in rope training is one of the tool's key differentiating factors.

Velocity is the speed at which an object travels. In this circumstance, the object is the battling rope. Without complicating things, 'velocity training' could be simply defined as training rope movements in either constant or changing patterns. When we perform movements with the rope, we refer to those movements as waves. 'Constant' means keeping the same speed when performing waves and 'changing' refers to increasing the speed or direction the wave travels.

In velocity training, you have the power going toward the anchor; as soon as the wave hits the anchor, there is feedback straight back to you. This challenges your stability.

There are different waves for different training outcomes:

- Waves for endurance – this refers to the aerobic conditioning that the rope can illicit in clients.

- Waves for power – the more power one produces, the greater the 'velocity effect', which is to say the force travelling to the anchor point returns with an equal and opposite reaction. When you perform a wave this way, there is greater power output and a greater level of stability required from the return of the force from the anchor point.

- Waves for speed – this targets the anaerobic system and creates a greater level of the lactate effect.

To gain the most out of the rope and achieve an incredible training effect, you want to get your clients tapping into endurance and speed drills while performing the waves.

- Endurance: Our goal is to perform waves non-stop for up to twenty minutes. I (Tarek) spent weeks preparing for the gruelling 20-minute level 2 John Brookfield battling ropes test. The process challenged me mentally and gave me a new level of endurance I had not experienced with running or other cardio activities. The cardio zone is achieved through sustaining sixty seconds or more of continuous activity. The intensity remains constant and consistent, in stark contrast to when we perform waves for speed. This is a whole-body movement, and the execution is fluid.

- Speed: Our goal here is to tap into the anaerobic system by doing short, fast and explosive sets. No longer than twenty seconds is advised. Greater body tension is required, and you will find that your core and arms work harder than when performing waves for endurance.

ONLINE RESOURCE: To view velocity training in action, visit our resource link – http://functionaltraininginstitute.com/book-resources/

Now we will look into the key rope movements in detail.

Progressions and complexes with the battling rope

KEY SAGITTAL MOVEMENTS

We begin in the sagittal plane for beginners primarily to establish the foundation of velocity training. By focusing on constant velocity, i.e. not changing direction into other planes, stability and endurance can be maintained and eventually mastered. Hence it is in the sagittal plane that mastery of the rope begins for all levels of client.

1. Double waves

The aim is to build up the level of endurance to five minutes and build up the technical proficiency which establishes the foundation to more complex movements with the rope.

By taking an extra step forward, the difficulty of the movement is increased. This is where a more advanced user would start.

Movement Execution

- Take hold of the battling rope, ensuring you do not have a tight grip as this will fatigue the forearm muscles
- Hinge slightly at the hips and start performing the wave movement from the hips, not the arms
- Keep the elbows pegged to the ribs as you move through the motions
- Remember to breathe in sequence: breathe in as the rope comes up and out as it comes down

Note: By using the hips, we become more efficient with the rope and therefore build up our levels of endurance. If the rope is performed with arms only, the arms will fatigue quickly.

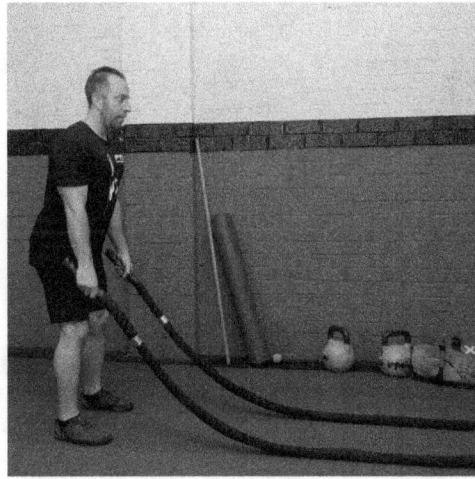
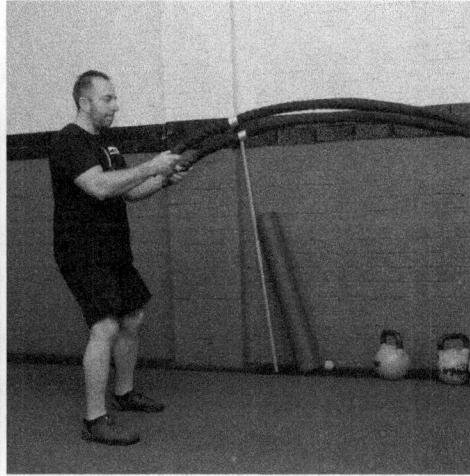

2. Walking version

The aim of this exercise depends on programming outcomes. A good place to start is to move through 4 steps, then reset. You can build your client's threshold quite easily and quickly this way. To progress the complex, perform 4 steps forward and instead of resetting, perform 4 steps backward to the start position.

Movement Execution

- Employ the rhythmic cue: 'Step and wave'
- Keep elbows from flaring out
- Take smaller steps
- Ensure lots of power from core and arms as you move through the steps

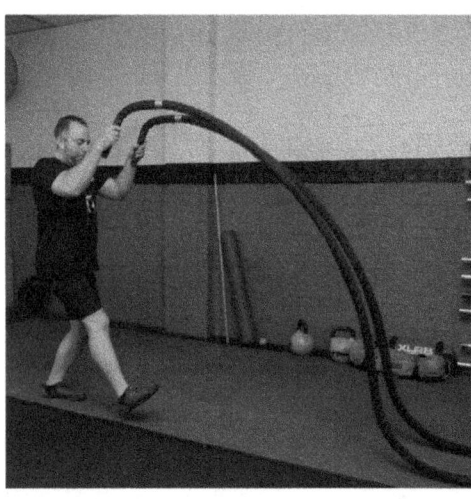
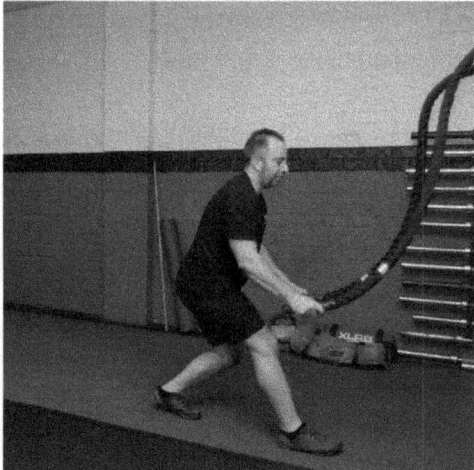

3. Kneeling

This is a harder movement to execute, so try not to spend a great deal of time performing from this position. Keep the trunk stable, but not so rigid that you cannot be fluid when performing the waves.

Movement Execution

- As with the standing position, hinge at the hips, keep the elbows in and begin the motion by driving from the hips
- As you move through the exercise, keep the toes pressed into the ground to increase stability
- Keep the breath cycles the same
- Keep the eyes on the anchor point

Note: Change the grips from classic (as shown in the picture) to neutral, where the thumbs are pointing up.

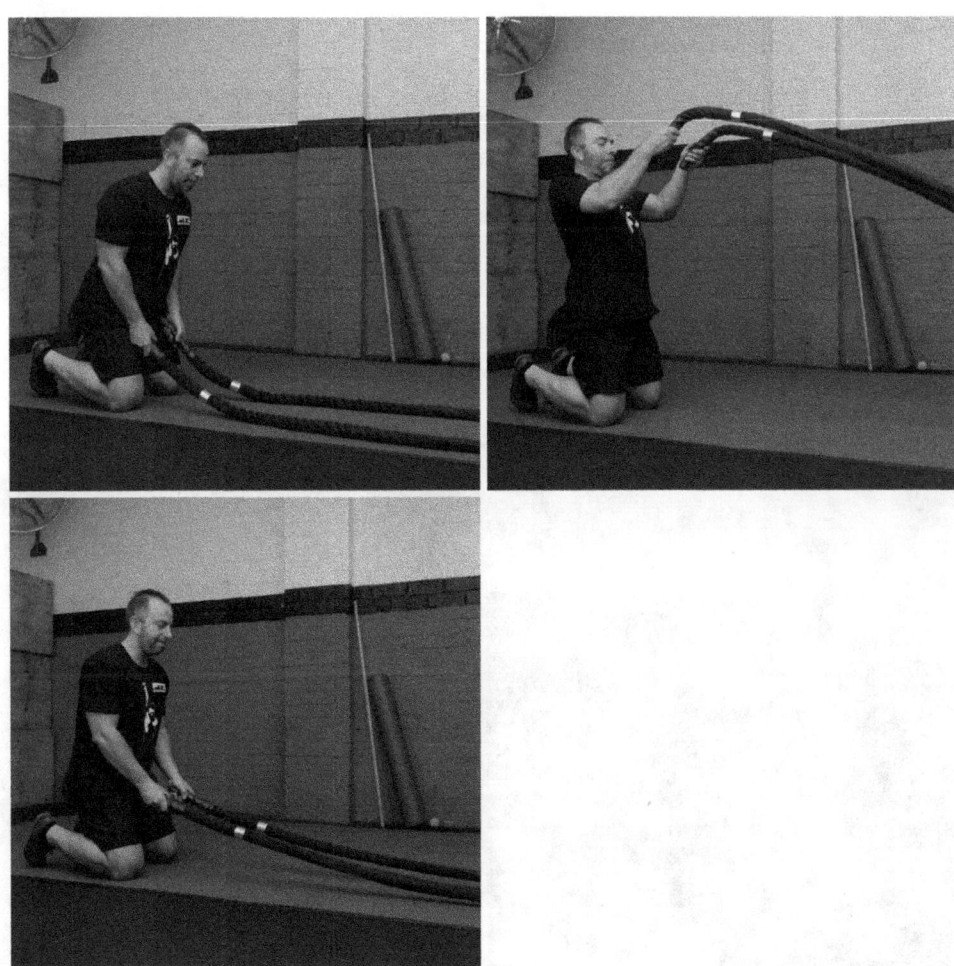

KEY TRANSVERSE MOVEMENTS

Once mastery is achieved in the sagittal plane, move on to the transverse-based movements. This is a great way to advance the complexity of the movement. By moving away from the sagittal and into the transverse, we begin to challenge stability, mobility and execution of the movement.

1. Bullwhip

The bullwhip has tremendous crossover to sport-based movements. It is an advanced movement, and clients will often compensate a lack of thoracic rotation by moving and rotating too much through the lumbar spine.

Movement Execution

- Pivot strongly by 'screwing the toes' into the ground
- Whip the rope from one side to the other, creating a semicircle shape
- As soon as the rope contacts the ground, transfer immediately to the next side
- Keep the waves smooth as you transition to each side
- Work strongly though the torso, performing as many smooth reps as possible

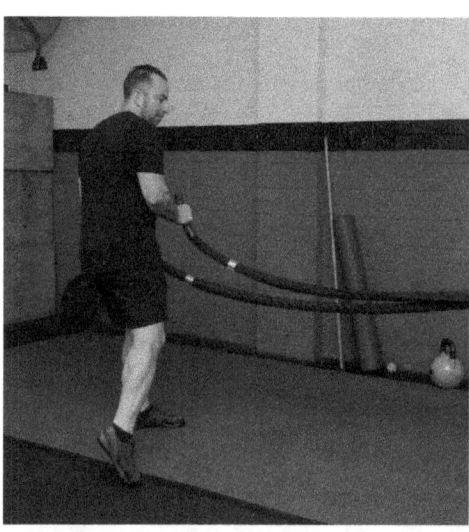
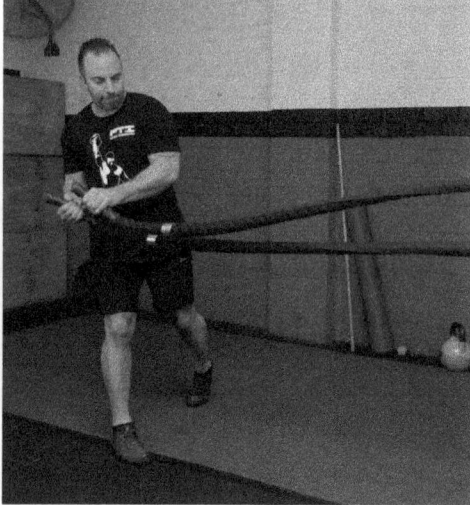

2. Rotational lunge switches

This is a more complex progression from the bullwhip. It involves an explosive lunge switch coupled with the exquisite timing of performing the wave.

Movement Execution

- Start by facing a 45-degree angle from the anchor (picture 1)
- Assume a lunge position – you will maintain this throughout the movement
- After performing a few reps, switch explosively to the opposite side (pictures 2 and 3)
- As you switch, keep the timing of the waves – maintain a sequence of switch and wave
- Start by doing 3 waves, then a switch
- As you get more accomplished, alternate 1 switch and 1 wave, with constant switches for time or repetition

Note: Try to land softly like a ninja as you switch.

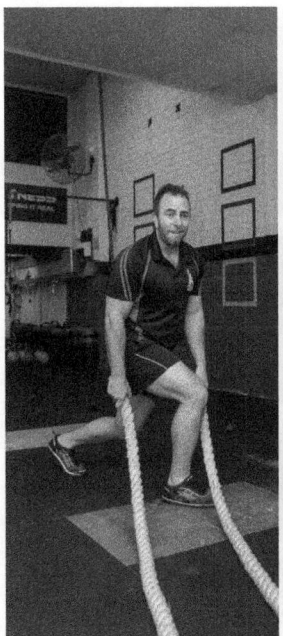 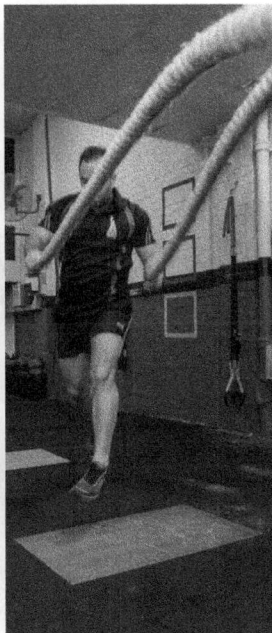 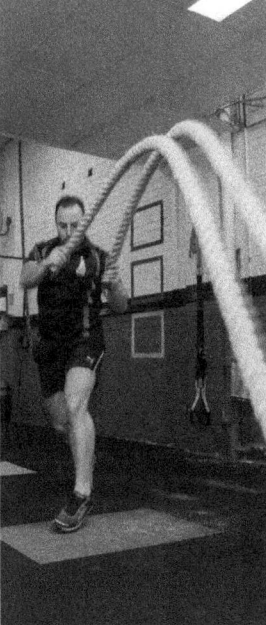

STRENGTH PULLS

The battling rope is very useful for pull-based exercises. These develop the pulling muscles of the body in a non-traditional way. Traditional ways of training centre on classic 'lever and load' movements that are fixed in the sagittal plane. We know that the body does not work in this one-dimensional way. We are designed to move three dimensionally, and our programming therefore needs to include the three planes of motion, sagittal, transverse and frontal, as well as movements that produce a combination of these. We have included a set of three-dimensional pulling exercises with the battling rope in order to develop greater levels of pulling and grip strength.

At FTI, the following exercises are considered critical to our programming. These positions can be performed either anchored or with a partner.

1. Standing pull (anchored)

Movement Execution

- With a strong neutral spine, reach and strongly pull
- Prevent the hips from rotating by anchoring the feet strongly into the ground
- Breathe in, then breathe out as you pull

Note: Engage the glutes and the posterior chain as you anchor your feet into ground, leading with the heel.

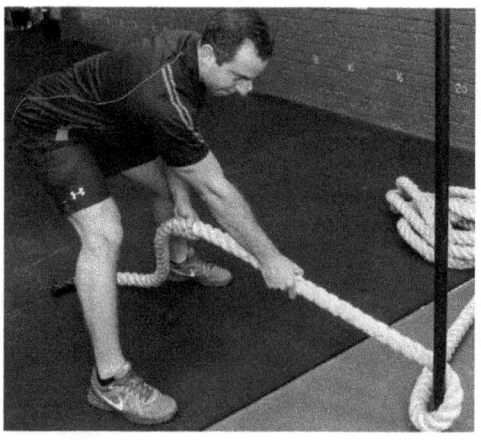

2. Seated pull (anchored)

Movement Execution

- Keep the trunk upright or slightly leaning back
- Dig the heels into the ground to anchor the lower body
- Keep the elbows in as you begin pulling
- After every 2 pulls, switch to the opposite side by pressing the rope above your head and onto the opposite shoulder

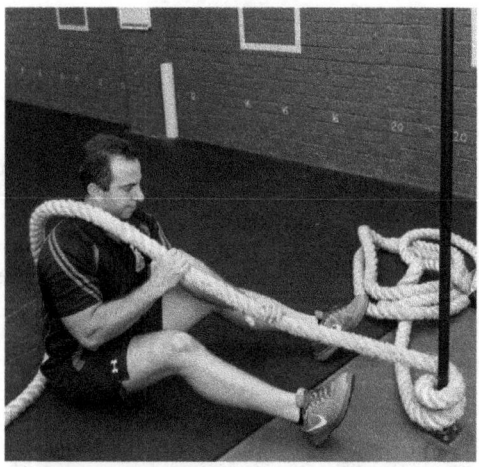

3. Side pull (anchored)

Movement Execution

- Begin with a flexed torso, keeping the spine neutral
- Pack the shoulders and begin pulling with the arm closest to the anchor point
- Avoid crossing the arms over as you continue to pull

Note: Remember to pull from both sides. You can also develop your weaker side by focusing a few more repetitions to that side.

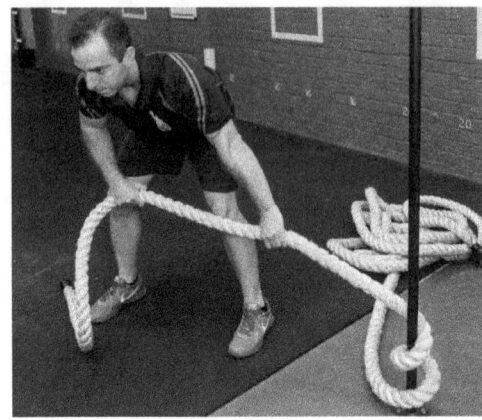

4. Kneeling pull (anchored)

Movement Execution

- From a kneeling position, begin your forward or side pulls
- Keep the trunk from collapsing as you pull
- There is greater emphasis on the core, so be active in the hips as you pull

Note: Keep a rhythm as you pull. By gaining momentum it will be easier to complete the cycle.

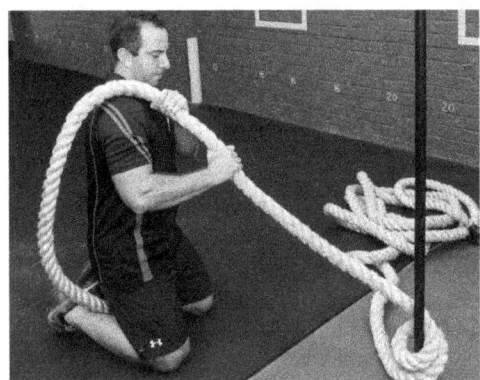

5. Partner pulls

If you do not have an anchor point for a rope, a partner can be the anchor. A coach can anchor a client, or you can pair off clients, with the added benefit of creating a sense of relatedness as they work out together.

These partner drills are challenging for both participants, as the person pulling is fighting the resistance offered by the anchoring partner, who in turn is challenged to stabilise and resist the pulling force. Here we have a classic case of opposing forces: Partner A resists and Partner B pulls against that resistance.

Try some of the following partner pull exercises:

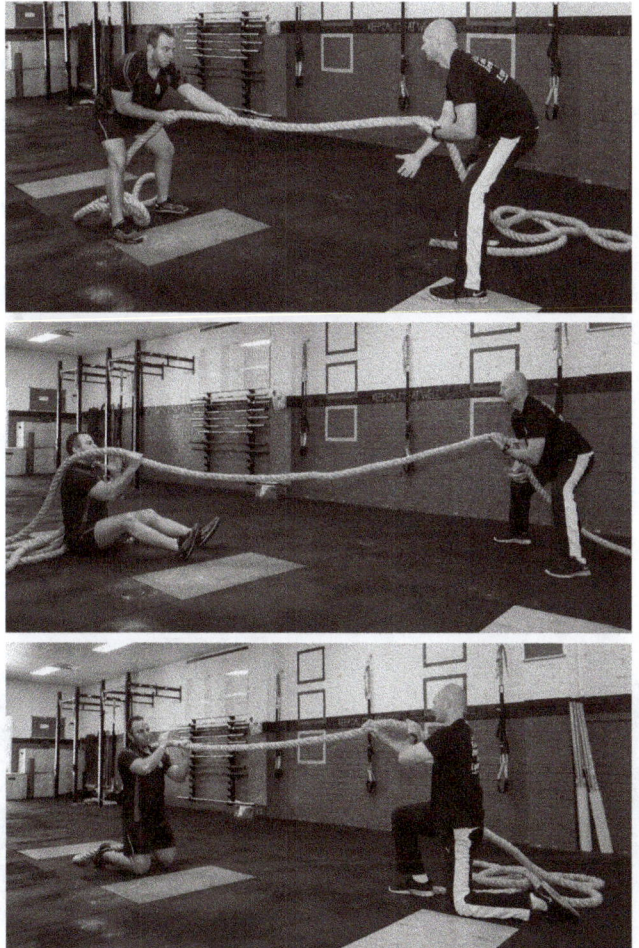

ONLINE RESOURCE: To watch the video about pulling-based movements visit – http://functionaltraininginstitute.com/book-resources/

KNEELING-TO-STANDING COMPLEX

Once we have become skilled in the velocity movements, we can string them together into a complex. The following exercise is an example of integrating complex patterns into one flowing movement which is made up of a series of three to five exercises.

This kneeling-to-standing complex is more dynamic and challenging than those performed with a weight held in front of the chest (like a medicine ball). It requires more control and coordination between upper and lower body. Therefore, this type of complex is what we would term a 'skill-based movement'. It is an excellent sequence for encouraging mastery and measuring progress in your client.

Note: This complex can be performed for time or reps. In this version, we stick with a 5-rep count for each movement, with the aim of building to 5 rounds of the complex.

Step 1 – Kneeling wave

Begin from a kneeling position. Perform 5 waves.

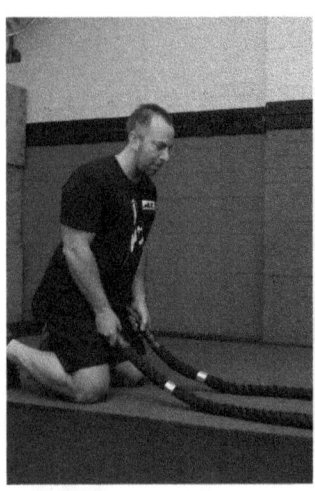 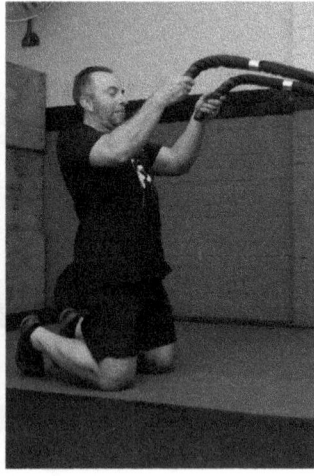 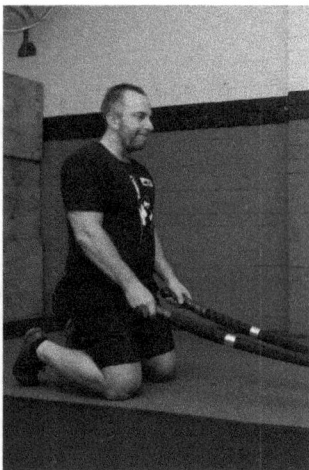

Step 2 – Half-kneeling wave

After the fifth wave, place one leg forward and perform 5 waves in this rested lunge position.

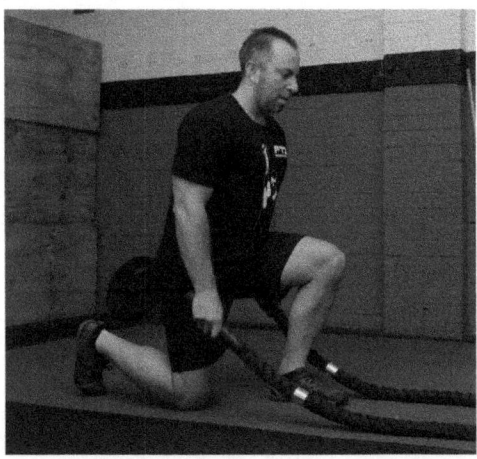

Step 3 – Standing wave

As you transition from step 2, push off to a standing postion and perform another 5 waves, this time standing.

Note: Make each transion smooth by keeping the waves flowing rather than stopping in between.

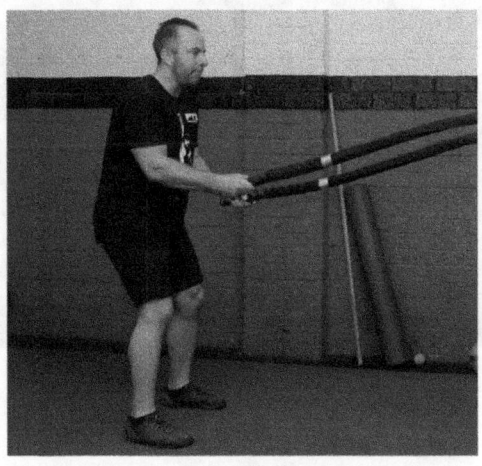

Step 4 – Reverse half-kneeling wave

After the fifth rep, Step back into resting lunge position, using the opposite leg from the one you used in step 2. Perform 5 waves here.

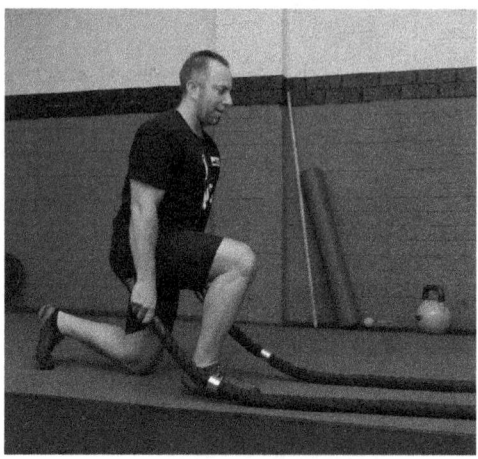

Step 5 – Back to kneeling wave

Finish in the kneeling position with 5 more waves.

Goal: Perform 5 continuous rounds of this complex.

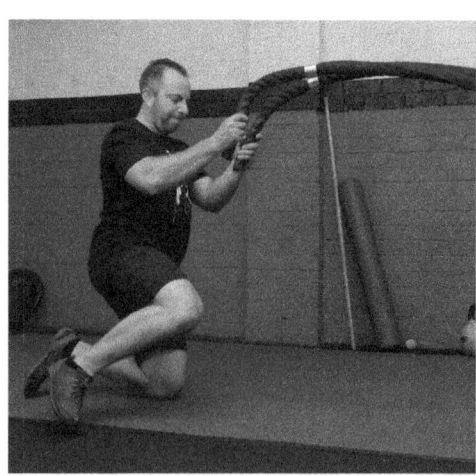
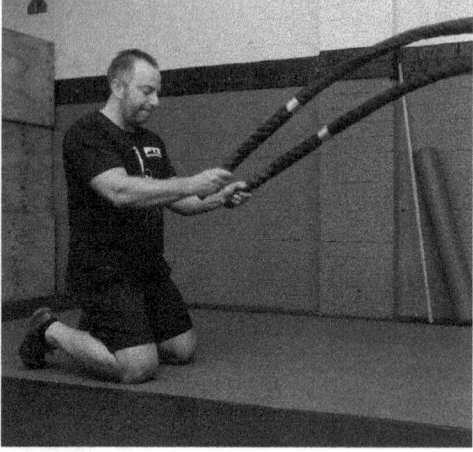

Complexes with other tools

As we have learned using the battling rope, a complex is a form of training that can be achieved using other tools or methods such as the kettlebell and functional bag. Integrating complex movement patterns is not beholden to one tool or method.

The tools we have selected are certainly not the only tools that can fit into the Adaptive FTS model. We can use barbells, mace clubs and torsion bars, to name just a few effective functional training tools and methods. Even Animal Flow® gets more complex, but only once the fundamentals have been mastered.

The following examples are ways in which those who go through the Adaptive FTS can begin fashioning programs that are more complex in nature.

TURKISH GET-UP (TGU)

Most people would think that the TGU is one exercise. At FTI we beg to differ. You are teaching your clients a movement complex that involves eight distinct steps, each requiring significant detail to ingrain correct execution. The level of coordination required is immense, and the extra emphasis on multiple movement patterns through the sequence equates to a complex.

- This is a grind-based movement; we recommend fewer reps
- Train the movements on both sides
- Learn the complex with bodyweight first, then increase the load progressively as you grow in strength and fluidity of movement
- Go through the movement slowly, using the breath to keep focused as well as maintaining eyes on the kettlebell for balance

Step 1 – Starting position

Movement Execution

- Safety roll into start position
- Roll to the side where the bell is and secure it before rolling onto your back
- Keep wrist straight and elbow 45 degrees off from the torso

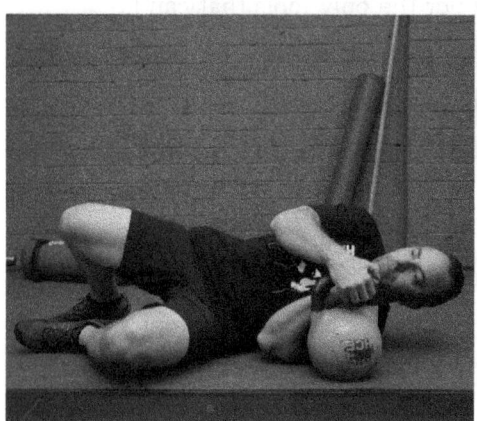 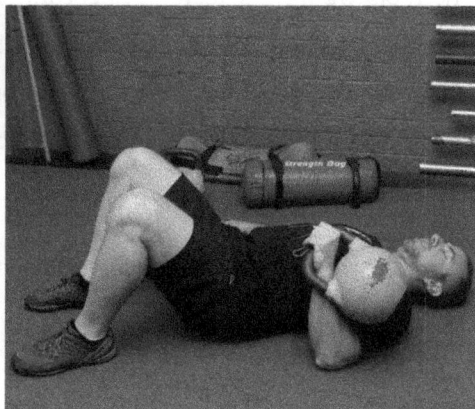

Step 2 – Press

Movement Execution

- Press feet and free arm strongly into the ground
- Slowly press the bell and keep it locked
- Keep wrist straight (picture 2)

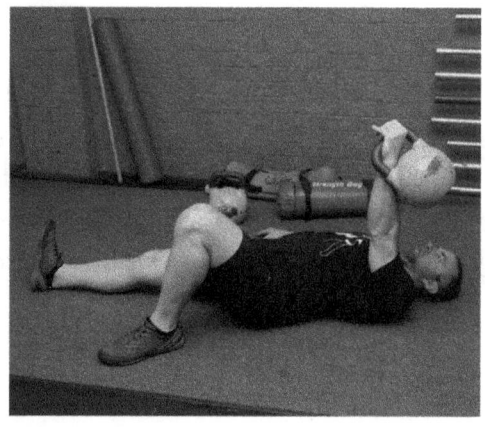

Step 3 – Drive to the opposite forearm

Movement Execution

- Drive powerfully toward the free arm
- Use the flexed leg (left in picture 3) and push off the foot to create effective leverage
- Keep eyes on the bell
- Maintain a strong lock-out position

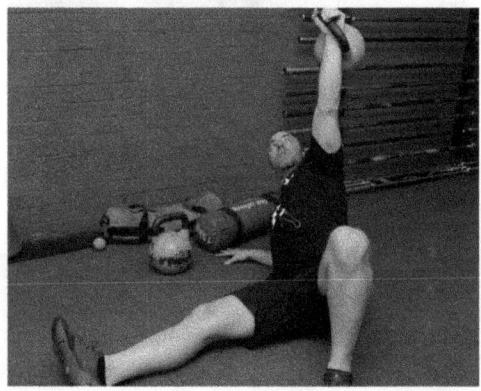

Step 4 – Hand transition

Movement Execution

- From the anchored forearm, push and screw the hand into the ground
- Make sure the shoulder, elbow and wrist are stacked
- Have the fingers pointing behind you to keep the shoulder externally rotated and in a secure position

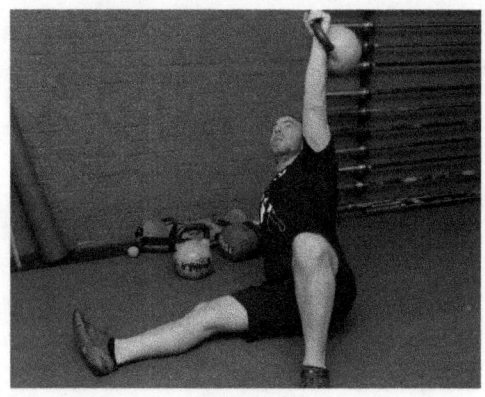

Step 5 – Bridge

Movement Execution

- Leveraging off the fixed hand and foot, drive the hips skyward
- Keep the eyes on the bell
- Keep pushing up, keeping the tension as you hold bridge position (picture 5)

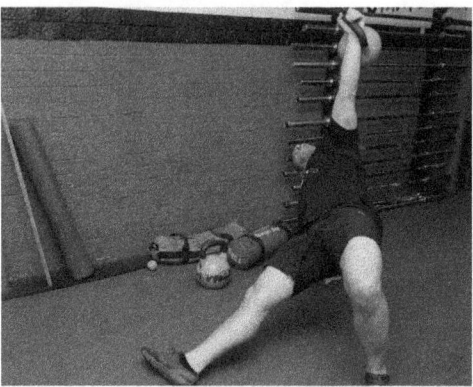

Step 6 – Side bend

Movement Execution

- Sweep the leg so that the knee sits between the fixed hand and foot (picture 6)
- Ensure the hips are not folded in but are pushed back – this will help create alignment and proper loaded positioning
- Make sure knee (left in picture 6) is in line with the ankle and foot

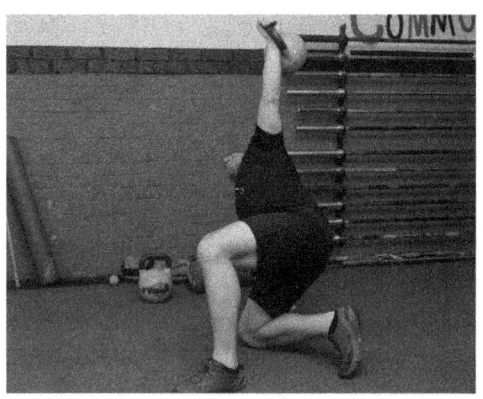

Step 7 – Lunge position

Movement Execution

- Phase 1: Push off the ground using the fixed hand and keep body upright (picture 7)
- Phase 2: Swivel the knee so we have a 90/90 set-up as in picture 8

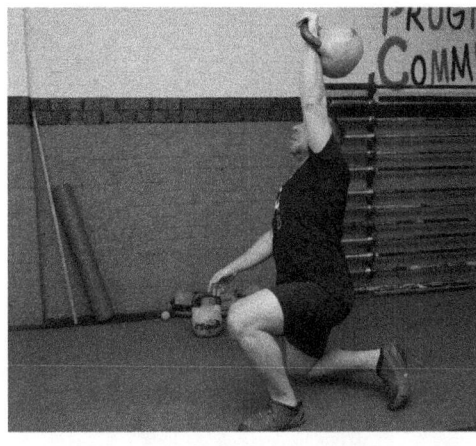
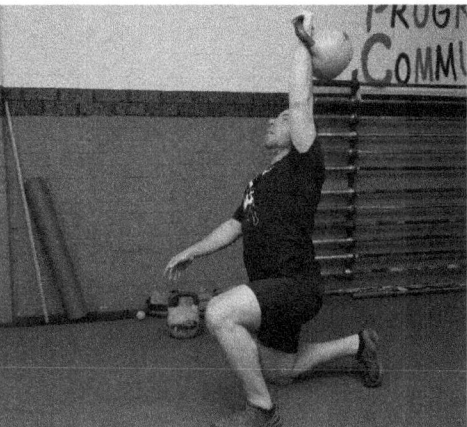

Step 8 – Standing

Movement Execution

- Push powerfully off the front foot to standing

Note: From the lunge position, the eyes can be adjusted to look toward the horizon. For beginners, it may be easier and provide more confidence intitally to keep the eyes on the bell.

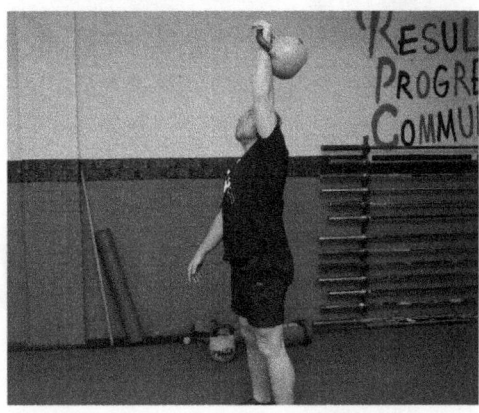

DOUBLE KETTLEBELL COMPLEX

This particular complex is for an advanced client who is well trained with the kettlebells. The complex combines four primal movement patterns: row, clean (hinge), squat and press. In such a complex, there is no room for sloppiness; the transitions are vital.

It is advised that you practise the single bell complex before trying this one.

Step 1 – Hinge ready position

Movement Execution

- Keep spine neutral and bend the knees
- Have shoulders and arms aligned above the bells
- Pull the shoulders into your 'back pockets'

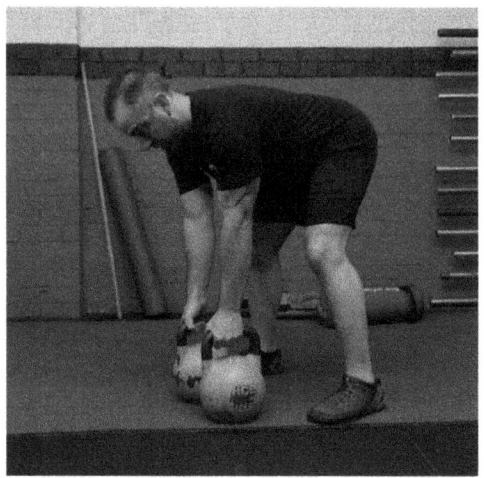

Step 2 – Perform a double bent over row

Movement Execution

- Strongly pull the bells toward your chest
- Slowly lower the bells back to start postion

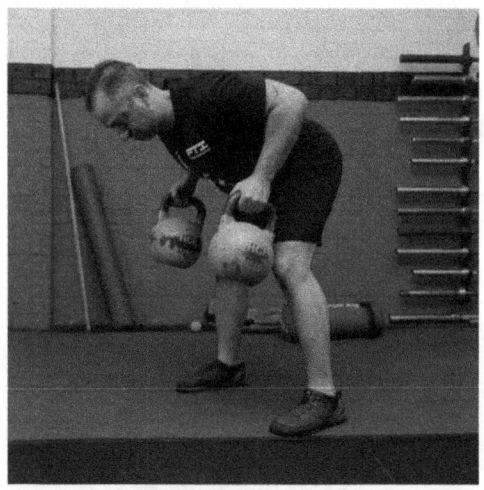

Step 3 – Reset into hinge ready position

Movement Execution

- Return to original position

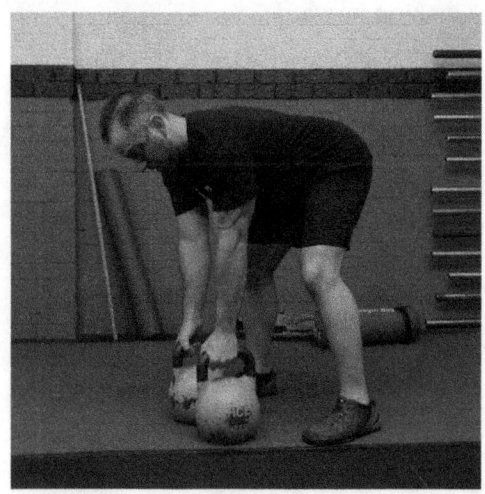

Step 4 – Clean the bells into rack position

Movement Execution

- Keep knees soft and trunk upright
- Look toward the horizon
- Relax the upper traps so you do not fatigue those muscles

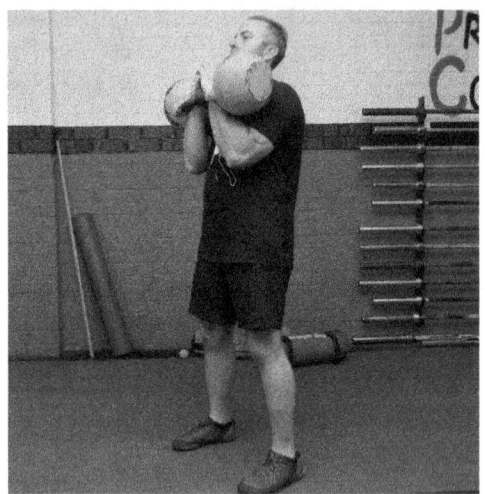

Step 5 – Perform a rack squat

Movement Execution

- Lower slowly into the squat, keeping the trunk upright
- Keep the eyes looking forward
- Pull the shoulders back to activate the backline

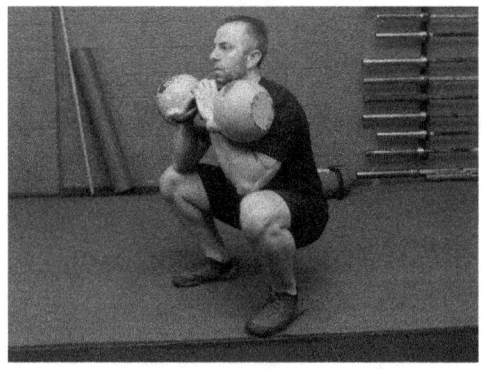

Step 6 – Perform a double press

Movement Execution

- From the squat position, power up into a double press
- Keep eyes looking forward
- Maintain a strong lock-out
- Bring the bells back to rack position to complete one round of the complex

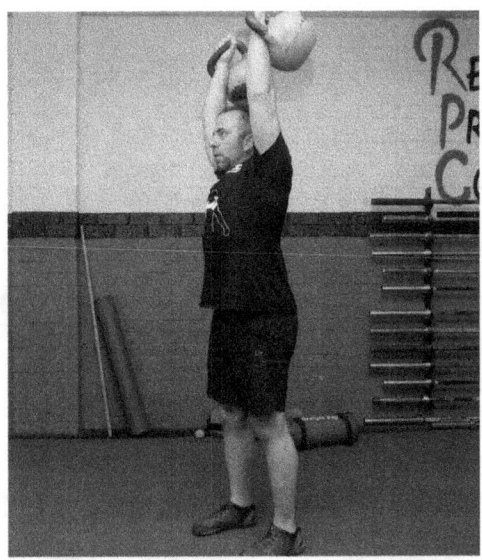

FUNCTIONAL BAG COMPLEX

This is the functional bag version of the double kettlebell complex. Using the bag for an identical complex is a way to regress the movement, provided the weight is not too dissimilar. It showcases the complementary nature of these two tools and systems.

Step 1 – Hinge ready position

Movement Execution

- Ensure the shoulders and entire arm are in alignment with the bag
- Keep a tall spine position
- Ensure bag is close to feet
- Slightly bend the knees to where the posture can be maintained

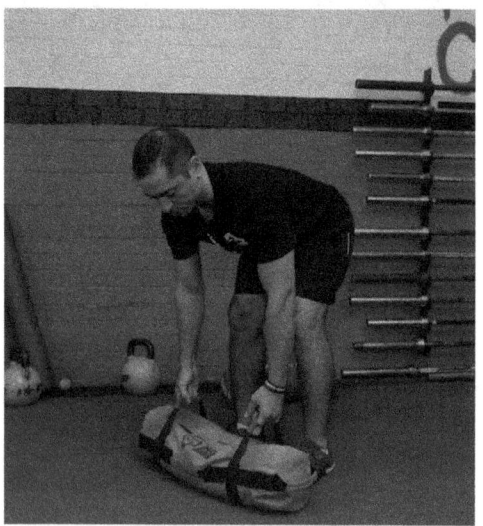

Step 2 – Perform a deadlift

Movement Execution

- Powerfully drive the bag up into standing position
- As you lift, pull the shoulders into the 'back pockets'
- Squeeze the glutes at the very top

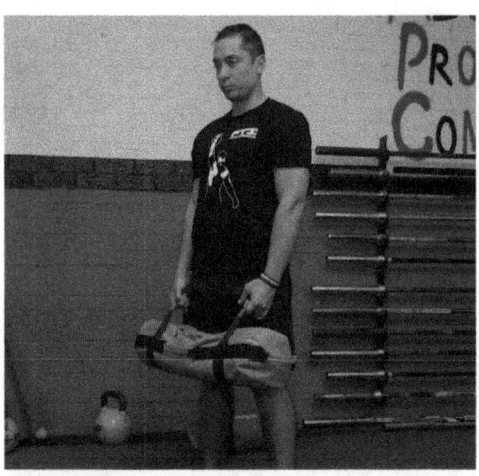

Step 3 – Set up in hang position

Movement Execution

- Slowly lower the bag into hang position, which is below the knees
- Adjust and maintain neutral spine

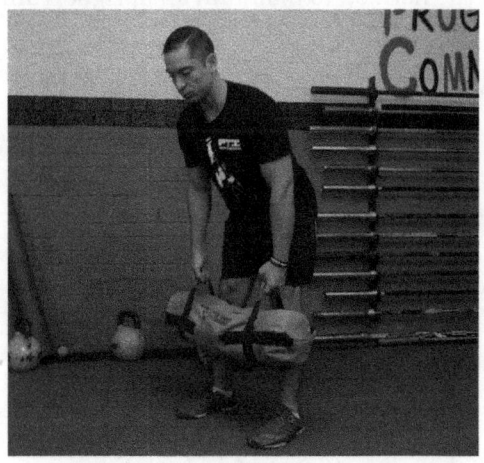

Step 4 – From hang position to clean

Movement Execution

- Explode the bag smoothly into rack position
- Ensure the bag contacts the shin and stays close to the midline of the body as it is pulled in to rack position

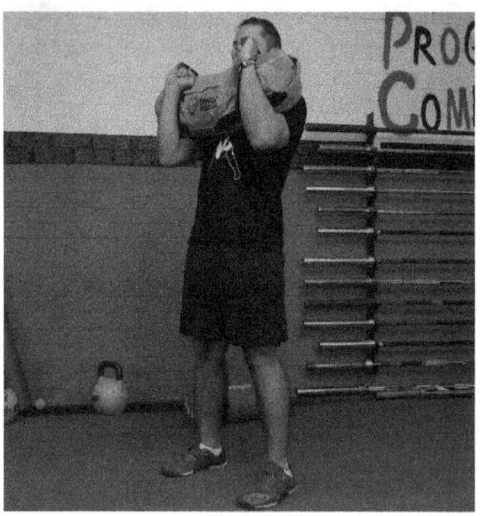

Step 5 – Perform a front squat

Movement Execution

- Keep bag hugged to chest as you squat
- Look toward the horizon to maintain an upright trunk

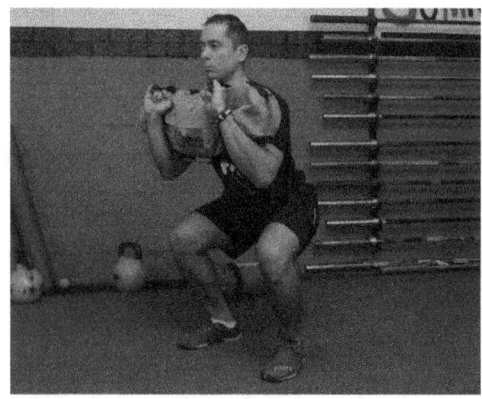

Step 6 – Perform a strict press

Movement Execution

- Complete the squat movement to standing before pressing
- Fully lock out the elbows and have the bag sit directly above your heels (picture 2)

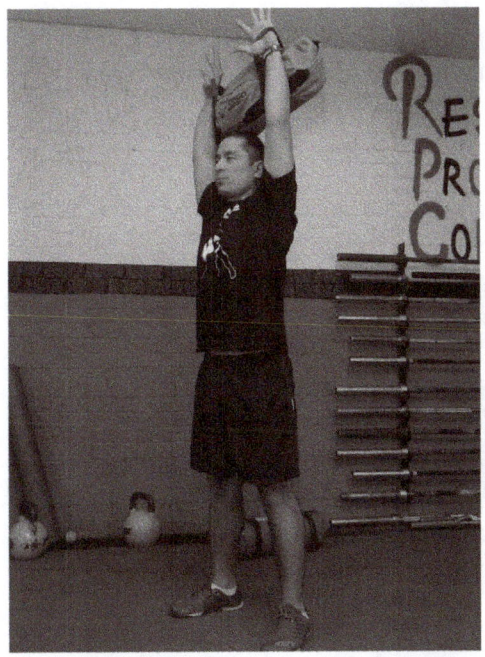

 ONLINE RESOURCE: To watch the instructional video compilation, visit – http://functionaltraininginstitute.com/book-resources/

Recap

Complex movement patterns can only be appreciated once the fundamentals are mastered. When the primary movement patterns are in place, however, there is great scope to layer in more sophisticated patterns – and to enjoy the training benefits.

The purpose of Pillar 5 is not just to showcase complex exercises, but to highlight the importance of progressions, variety and creativity in programming in order to encourage skill acquisition and mastery in your client. As you have seen, this can be done with a variety of tools.

The battling rope is a fantastic tool with which to explore and exploit the complexity of velocity training. Through challenging the stability of the body with a dynamic force while simultaneously requiring the endurance of maintaining waves, the rope poses an immediate challenge for any client. Additionally, the integration of unconventional pulling movements not only brings about more functional strength, but also places a new neural demand on anyone new to the rope and this unique training system.

Part 4: Program with Purpose

Bringing It All Together

Programming Theory: Behind the Adaptive FTS

Now it's time to show you how to build programs for your clients based on the 5 Pillars of Functional Training.

The Adaptive FTS approach to programming is unique, because it presents a personalised, progressive and systematic way to take clients from A to Z. This is not a magic formula for the coach to simply plug in. Every client who walks in the door will have different needs. Our approach to programming is adaptive in that it is not simply linear, nor is it random or full of second-guessing. It is a fluid, dynamic and thoughtful system that provides structure, requiring the coach to think outside the box. Successful programming lies in all that has come before it: solid coaching fundamentals and techniques, skills in assessing and preventing injury and, of course, deep understanding of the functional movements themselves, as covered in Parts 1, 2 and 3 of this book. Without this foundation, programming loses the power to truly transform clients from the inside out.

Our programming style is based on the principle of periodisation, but incorporates our pillars in order to produce an adaptive program for a wide range of clients and goals. In this chapter, we first unpack our take on periodisation. We then take a look at the three levels of programming that go into building a periodised program:

- The macrocycle or training plan
- The mesocycle or training phases
- The microcycle or individual sessions

Finally, we will consider the importance of reviewing your programming.

Understanding periodisation

To periodise or not to periodise? The word 'periodisation' is tossed around a bit in fitness circles, so it's worth asking questions about what it is, whether it's necessary and how to apply it to a broad range of clients.

Periodisation means the subdivision (or 'chunking down') of a training plan. This style of systematic planning for athletic or physical training was originally developed for competitive athletes (and successfully validated by the Russians during the 1960 Olympic games).

The benefit of periodising is that client goals can be measured and achieved by following a plan. With all goals in life, we are taught to break them down into small, achievable chunks. The same applies when training clients, whether recreational fitness enthusiasts or athletes. We simply break the long-term physical training goal of our client into smaller and more achievable chunks. It can certainly be applied to anyone wanting to reach their physical potential. That plan may be three months, six months or whatever length of time you set for your client's 'big goal'. It allows the coach to plan big and make training more like a journey for the client, with opportunities to build and experience results at each stage, achieving a sense of success for both coach and client.

Logical Sequence of Training diagram

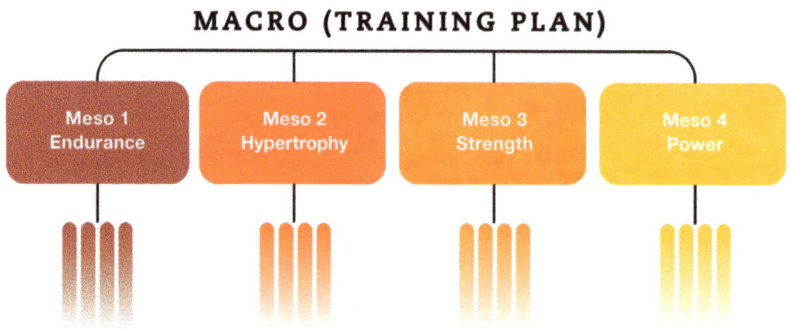

The diagram shows what is known as a 'logical sequence of training'. Endurance comes before hypertrophy, hypertrophy comes before strength and strength comes before power. This is indeed logical for many athletic applications, and is recognised by strength and conditioning coaches who are preparing athletes for competition. In Meso1, for example, the focus would be on improving the endurance training qualities. Athletes would still be training the other qualities such as strength and power, but with a low portion of the training time, as the predominant goal for that cycle is to develop endurance.

Periodisation is widely used in strength and conditioning circles in this way. Quite often, however, the language we employ to devise our periodised systems can become a stumbling block for us and our clients. When we fixate on macro, meso and microcycles and a rigid order of endurance, hypertrophy, strength and so on, we can become inflexible in our programming content, not to mention confusing for our non-athlete clients, who may not know what to do with such technical ideas.

Another important issue to ponder is how well a long-term periodised program can be managed and maintained, especially for the general fitness client. Training may get interrupted by illness, a holiday or a busy patch at work. This is life, right? How can we as coaches best navigate this tricky terrain?

Let's rethink the system. An adaptive system is one that employs phases such as hypertrophy, fat loss, rehab and so forth, but in a more fluid and flexible way. It tracks and measures clients through their different phases yet is responsive to the dynamics of daily life mentioned above. If a client is progressing through a phase and then happens to miss a week or even more, when they return they can simply pick up where they left off or potentially regress to the previous phase.

Our view at FTI is that because our general clients are not professional athletes, adaptive periodising is essential. Being flexible to the needs of the client is part of the skill of the coach. With the Adaptive FTS, the client is still on some phase of training and there is clear, progressive method. Our phases, while not the traditional mesocycles, are still essentially periodised mesocycles, as they remain within a system of planning and progression. As personal trainers, while we may not be preparing athletes for competition we still need to follow a 'logical sequence of training'. This is where the 5 Pillars come into play.

In the following diagram, we have replaced the meso phases with the pillars.

Logical Sequence of Training with 5 Pillars diagram

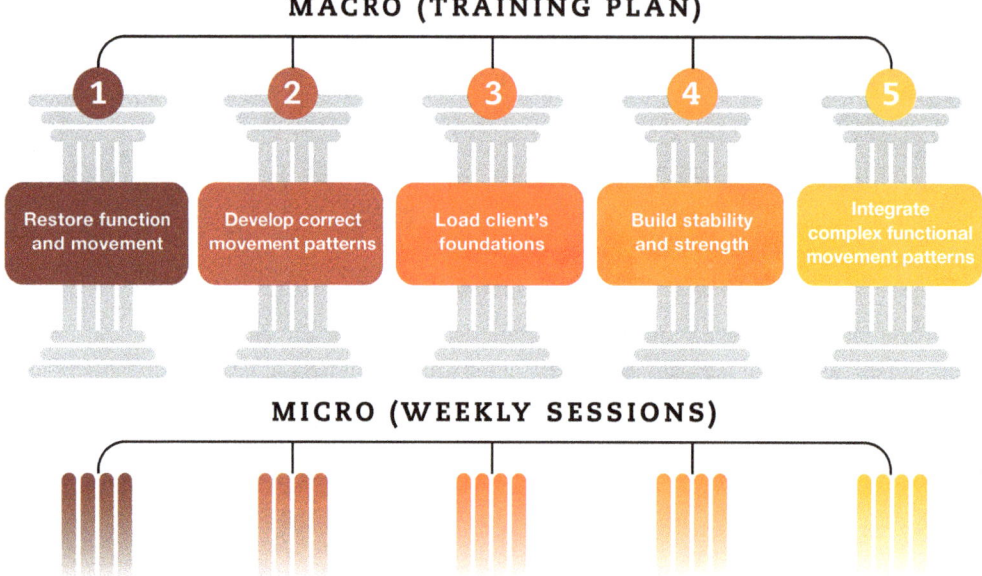

Where a client will start and how long they will spend in each phase depends on where they may be on the exercise continuum. For example, a client who presents with very little training history and has mobility issues will spend more time in Pillar 1. Many factors will influence the decision about how long to spend in the phase, including training frequency, age, training intent, injury history, training age, mindset, motivation, nutrition and lifestyle. This is why assessing, not guessing, is of paramount importance to the coach.

As mentioned earlier, each phase of training represents the objective or target training quality that you are aiming to achieve for that cycle. However, it does not mean it is the sole focus. If a client needs to restore function of their shoulders, for example, you can still work on their movement in that region (Pillars 1 and 2) while helping them to build up their endurance and strength (Pillars 3 to 5).

The names we have given the pillars (for example, 'Restore function and movement') will help clients to understand the purpose of the training phases you set for them. However, they will understand it even better if you refine your phase names to align with specific outcomes and other milestone objectives, such as:

1. Improve shoulder mobility and develop proper movements
2. Improve cardiovascular endurance and flexibility
3. Lose fat and build muscle
4. Focus on strength

Variety is also a key, and mesocycles can be interchanged for other goals that are novel, such as:

1. Eight-week fat loss challenge (eight-week mesocycle)
2. Charity runs
3. Spartan obstacle course training

This will add greater drive and purpose to their journey. As we discussed in Part 1, *Coach with Purpose*, incorporating the 'why' behind what they are doing will increase the client's engagement and participation levels, ensuring consistency, which is the bedrock of success for any training plan.

We will now take a closer look at some of the things you need to consider at each level of periodised programming.

The macrocycle/training plan

When creating a functional training program, you first need to create an overarching training plan. We call this the macrocycle. The length of a macrocycle depends on the goals of the client. If you have established a three-month time frame to get a client into shape for their wedding, for example, then that three months is the macrocycle. It is client-dependent, and that is both the beauty and challenge of programming.

A powerful way to approach your macrocycle planning is with FTI's 'five layers of successful programming', which will help you to think clearly about the purpose of a particular macrocycle for your client.

FIVE LAYERS OF SUCCESSFUL PROGRAMMING

1. Clarify client goal

To set up our client for success, we need to find out their short and long-term goals. More importantly, we want to discover their *qualitative* goals. It is easy for us to fixate on measuring quantifiable goals (like skill improvement, fat loss or a strength target). As necessary as it is to set these goals and measure the results, we'll program most successfully by working with the client to discover what it is they really want out of this training. Let me give you an example:

> Many years ago at the gym I owned, Primal NRG Fitness in Sydney, Christine came to me quite broken in confidence. She had not trained for many years. Her physiological measures were poor, even to a point where she could not row 100 metres without puffing away and giving up. After taking her through a comprehensive **assessment**, we established the usual and obvious goals for a three-month time frame: improve her cardio, with a goal to row 1,000 metres continuously;

lose body fat by 10%; and be able to perform a 20kg loaded squat. As great as these were for her, as we began the training and trust was built between us, Christine opened up about her desire to climb Machu Pichu. And there it was! The actual qualitative and deeper goal for Christine was to eventually climb the mountain. We altered her programming slightly into training phases, and twelve months later Christine sent me and my business partner Ray a photo of herself atop the magnificent Machu Pichu.

2. Clarify client level

You will have clients walk in your door from all kinds of backgrounds and with unique experiences and circumstances. Yes, each and every one of your clients is just like you and me. There are the training histories, past injuries and body types to contend with. Profiling your client and understanding where their journey begins will set you and the client up for success. Let's look at another example:

> Michael has not trained for five years, apart from his incidental fifteen minutes a day of walking to work and back. He has only played sport at school level and now, at forty years of age, wants to get in shape again. You also discover that he has poor overall mobility. Where do you think Michael will begin the journey according to the Adaptive FTS? It's safe to say, right at the beginning – Pillar 1: Restore function and movement.

3. Clarify client style/preference

As we have identified in Part 1, *Coach with Purpose*, personality profiling will help us to determine what the client's preferences and style are so we can truly personalise and then customise their training plan. We all have preferences. You will recall the idea of self-determination, in which there is always a balance between the 'control of the coach' and the 'autonomy of the client'. Instead of having a fixed and rigid session plan, incorporate some flexibility into your macrocycle. This means, for example, giving the client equipment options (functional bag or kettlebell?) yet keeping the same movement. Or changing the environmental stimulus by training in a different part of the gym or going outdoors. You may also have a couple of different program types and ask, 'Which one would you like to choose today?' The guile in this is that both programs will have the same training load, yet you have managed to increase client autonomy by adding choice.

4. Training plan

Based on the above, we can then begin to construct the periodised plan that will take your client on a journey that is based on experience, progress and results.

5. Assess and review

Clients experience many barriers that can prevent them from sticking to their training programs. Unfortunately, trainers often don't devote much time to prepare for this. There needs to be give and take on both sides, so you need to allow a bit more flexibility when working with 'non-professional' athletes. It is your job to factor in your client's lifestyle when preparing their program.

Therefore, as you decide what goals to set at a macrocycle level in your programming, it is imperative that you take into account your client's personal circumstances and mindset as well as their physical capabilities. In the assessment phase you will need to identify what it is exactly that your client is able to do – and what it is that they are willing to commit to. The mindset and coaching component of the Adaptive FTS will play a huge part in empowering your clients.

Progressing a client or athlete through a functional training program safely and efficiently requires clear understanding of an individual's prior training and exercise history. This then allows you to understand the client's training capabilities. Information such as the type and length of prior and technical lifting proficiency should all be recorded before commencing a functional training program. Training intensity and frequency is then decided based on the client's current training status.

The mesocycle/training phase

Once the training plan is established with your client, then it is a case of breaking the macro goal into achievable and relevant phases. When matching a client's long-term goal with their macrocycle, there are any number of different phases (mesocycles) that we could look to incorporate: fat loss, general physical preparedness, energy systems training and so forth.

Within the Adaptive FTS model, the pillars can be phased this way:

- Mesocycle/Phase 1: Restore function and develop proper movement patterns (Pillars 1 and 2)
- Mesocycle/Phase 2: Development of foundational strength and stability (Pillar 3)
- Mesocycle/Phase 3: Layer in advanced strength and power (Pillar 4)
- Mesocycle/Phase 4: Integrate complex movement sequencing (Pillar 5)

The length of each phase is determined by the training plan. If your client can only train two times per week, then your phase may be eight weeks long. On the other hand, if your client can train four times per week, then that phase may take four weeks to achieve. This is where you as the coach must be adaptive and create the phases around the client, not the other way around. Your periodised training plan is a map; it is a living guide that is malleable to your client's individual circumstances.

Bear in mind that the Adaptive FTS is designed such that you may have clients who accelerate through the system. Well-trained clients may begin at Pillar 4, for example, incorporating what is necessary from earlier pillars as they go.

Another thing to note with the system is that each pillar can be broken into multiple phases. For example, Pillar 2 (developing proper movement patterns) may be broken into:

- Phase 1 – Coordination and stability (duration 4 weeks)
- Phase 2 – Lower body conditioning (4 weeks)
- Phase 3 – Upper body conditioning (4 weeks)

The microcycle/sessions

Microcycles are essentially the individual sessions in a given week. You might prepare four to six weeks within a mesocycle.

First of all, you need to determine training frequency (how many sessions per week). Ideally, you will have your client committed to a minimum of four sessions per week. This can be two with you and two on their own. The challenge here is ensuring that these sessions are monitored and measured. A suggestion here is to get them a diary to monitor the progress of their sessions. Without tracking sessions, your training phase will be inaccurate.

At FTI we believe strongly in empowering your clients. In order to effect this, let's take a look at a simple but extremely effective method in ensuring the success of your training plan. The more someone trains, the better, because the faster they will adapt to the training quality they are targeting. Four sessions per week is an achievable target for most people, and a volume that produces proven results – provided the sessions are of good quality and involve enough challenge to elicit the outcomes you are aiming for.

PROGRAMMING TYPES

A key element of smart and sustained session programming is variability. The body responds best to varied stimulus, and changing up programming methods is a sure way of achieving this. To reduce boredom and stagnation, the coach must be familiar with different programming types, from anaerobic to endurance to strength.

There are myriad ways a coach can program for a session, including periodising a mixture of types. Here are a few methods we like to incorporate into our structured programming:

AMRAPS (As Many Rounds as Possible)

We can take metabolic conditioning (met-con) or high intensity training into what is called AMRAPS (commonly used in CrossFit training). The AMRAPS session includes a cardio/aerobic exercise, anaerobic exercise and a combination of different movement patterns, such as including unilateral or asymmetrical loading with some of the exercise selections.

Trainers can expect many benefits when instructing clients with AMRAPS. There will be measurable metabolic/neural conditioning improvement, provided form is not compromised and movements are executed with proper technique. Other physiological benefits include increased EPOC (Exercise Post Oxygen Consumption) and positive hormonal excretions (growth hormone and testosterone). What's more, programming for time may be a better method of managing groups where the physical demographics vary: you may have a beginner client who completes a simpler, less intense workout than the more experienced campaigner who wants to be pushed. Therefore, the principles of progression and overload can be factored in to cater for different fitness levels.

Some risks of training with AMRAPS include compromised form/technique at the expense of 'getting it done', inadequate recovery time leading to neural fatigue and poor mechanical compensations (bad form), dangerously high lactate levels in less conditioned clients and the possibility of overtraining due to too many intense sessions without adequate rest programmed in.

Tabata programs

One form of HIIT, which started as a metabolic conditioning exercise in a controlled environment and has been shown to be effective for met-con, is Tabata training. This form of programming has been popularised and has morphed into a way of incorporating time-based interval training along the lines of high intensity.

Note: FTI's Tabata protocol is not met-con in its truest sense: instead, it is a way to keep intensity levels high while adding rest periods after each round. (A round is 4 minutes long and 8 cycles of 20 seconds work and 10 seconds rest). Rest is a necessity for the beginner and is typically scheduled after each round. In order for your client to successfully complete another cycle, they need to recover all lost energy. Training adaptations require a proper work-to-rest ratio. For a beginner, rest after one full round should be at least four minutes. So, your thirty-minute workout for a beginner may initially be limited to three rounds.

Complexes

In our programming at FTI, we place significant emphasis on complexes. As we've discussed in Part 3, complexes are a great way to take fundamental movement patterns and work them into fun, challenging and dynamic workouts.

World-renowned functional training expert and author of the book *The New Rules of Lifting*, Alwyn Cosgrove, describes the three key features that make a movement pattern a complex:

1. Use of one tool (for example, a kettlebell)
2. Performed in a small space
3. Use of at least three movement patterns

At FTI, you will see these three features in our complexes. Refer to the complexes in Pillar 5 for some great complexes to get you started.

Challenges

Challenges are a great way to motivate clients and instil a sense of achievement – and help ensure they return. The key is to link challenges with two tangibles:

1. Progress
2. Results

Clients will continually return to your sessions only if they see sufficient progress and results. If they are insufficiently challenged, they are unlikely to achieve a sense of accomplishment or flow and are likely to develop false theories as to why their training lacks consistency. They may stagnate or simply cease training altogether.

Challenges must be a balance of anticipation and competition: they need to be tough enough for the clients to get excited about challenging themselves and progressing, but not so challenging that they cause fear and dread of what is to come. Deep down, everyone wants to know how far they have come. It's a key factor in the drive and determination to overcome challenges in the first place.

At FTI we recommend incorporating challenges after each mesocycle/training phase to provide the quantifiable progress your clients may be yearning for. Incorporating challenges at this point also serves as a way to progress your client and ensure they 'earn the right' to begin the next training phase.

PRINCIPLES FOR ADAPTIVE SESSION PROGRAMMING

All sessions we design and deliver are about an **experience**. Therefore, how much energy we provide in the session (engagement, encouragement and empowerment) will determine the success of the session. There are occasions when the coach needs to adapt to unforeseen circumstances when the client shows up. Perhaps they have come in a few minutes late. Will you compromise some of the warm-up or reduce the main part of the workout? A client may come in a little run down. Will you reduce the intensity of the session so as not to tip them over the edge and have them truly run down? A client walks in highly stressed and needs to vent some anger. How would you manage that? These challenges exist, and it is up to the coach to be adaptive in their approach.

What's more, our sessions need to be tailored to the client. Here are some of the principles that will help you to plan your programs well – and adapt in the moment when needed.

Principle of load

Load is the appropriate dose you give each of the clients in the group. In their book *Principles and Practice of Resistance Training*, Stone and Sands relate how vital it is for the coach to plan and implement ever-increasing demands, and that improvement can occur only when training loads are above average and the athlete/client must dip into adaptation reserves, i.e. the client is stressed and the body must respond by adapting to the new stress.[66]

Providing a selection of loaded tools (such as functional bags and kettlebells) ensures clients will not be caught in the 'comfortable workout' trap. The aim is to challenge the group as a whole by challenging each client enough to elicit the requisite stimulus and training effect.

---

66   Michael Stone, Margaret Stone and William Sands, *Principles and Practice of Resistance Training*, Champaign US, Human Kinetics, 2007.

Training load is not just about how much weight a client can lift. It considers two key factors:

- Volume: work capacity, for example, 'Is the client able to complete a five-minute battling rope set?'

- Intensity: complexity of a given exercise or changed variables within a program. For example, doing eight kettlebell presses a minute instead of seven increases the workout intensity and decreases the resting time.

Gear system	HR Max (heart rate)	Difficulty	RPE (Rate perceived ex)
1	50–60% of Max	Easy	0–2
2	60–70% of Max	Somewhat Easy	2–4
3	70–80% of Max	Moderate to Somewhat hard	4–6
4	80–90% of Max	Hard	6–8
5	90–100% of Max	Very Hard	8–10

Relevant here is what PTA Global calls 'training in gears'.[67] Intensity may need to be changed on a given day based on the external circumstances (things that are out of your hands) such as a niggly injury (back to restoring function and movement), a cold or the client's level of stress. How well are you in tune with the body language of your client?

Progressions and regressions

Programs lacking progressions will lead to group stagnation and boredom. On the other hand, programs must also offer exercise regressions to allow struggling clients to remain motivated to finish the exercise – and the program.

How to ensure an exercise and program are readily modifiable for the 'less experienced' client? By developing a list of exercises with appropriate

---

67   Read more here: www.ptacademy.edu.au/what-gear-do-you-drive-your-clients-in/

progressions and regressions, which is what we have done for you with the FTI Programming Continuum.

Programming continuum

Hinge	Powerbag Kneeling Deadlift Series	PB Standing Deadlift Series	Romanian Deadlift	Kettleball Swing	Double Kettleball Swing	Battling Rope High Wave
Press	Powerbag Press (Vertical Hold)	Kettlebell Supine Press	Suspension Training Chest Press	Kettlebell See-saw Press	BB Shoulder Press	Kettlebell Reverse Grip Press
Row	Kettlebell Bent Over Row With Irradiation	Kettlebell Split Stance Bent Over Row	Suspension Trainer Row	BB Bent Over Row	Battling Rope Strong Man Pulls	Kettlebell Renegade Row
Core	Kettlebell Single-leg Bilateral Deadlift	Kettlebell Halo	Kettlebell Rack Position Walking	Kettlebell Offset Carry	Suspension Trainer Pike	Turkish Get-up
Squat	Suspension Trainer Squat	Powerbag Zercher Squat	Kettlebell Offset Squat	Powerbag Overhead Squat	BB Back Squat	Kb Pistol Squat

As you can see, this is not an exhaustive list of exercises. As you compile more functional exercises for your programs, you will need to strip the exercise down and ensure you have progressions and regressions in place. For example, an exercise involving multiple movement patterns and planes of motion should be classified as a complex movement requiring regressions. The table provided is a great example of a straightforward exercise continuum using some of our favourite functional tools, which can serve as an aid to the coach to ensure movement progression.

Principle of variety

The key to any successful, sustainable program is to prevent boredom and stagnation by changing things up with a variety of exercises coupled with a progressive program. As Zatsiorsky and Kraemer discuss in their remarkable book, *Science and Practice of Strength Training*, adaptation means the adjustment of an organism (client) to its environment (program). If the environment (program) changes, the organism (client) changes to better survive (training stressors) the new conditions (training outcomes).[68]

Specificity principle

The principle of specificity is summarised by the acronym 'SAID', which stands for Specific Adaptations to Imposed Demands. If the goal of your client is to perform 100 kettlebell swings in five minutes, then the load of the kettlebell and the variable of time acting as volume need to be realistic to this goal. The 'imposed demands' of reaching 100 swings in five minutes must be adequately met with lighter loads, less time and proper technique first and foremost.

Specificity may be described in another way, as a principle of 'transfer of training results'. Will a high volume of swings transfer well to the kettlebell snatch? Or will 100 double rope waves be just as effective? Even though there is no scientific study to validate this, the action of the one-arm swing is a precursor to the kettlebell snatch in learning inertia and the momentum of the kettlebell. The waves may help, but the transferability of the one-arm swing is far superior.

Complexity and skill acquisition

Complexity is a key ingredient in eliciting cumulative training effects. First, client consistency is an important determinant in whether a coach should add more difficult and challenging exercises. A client must have demonstrated sufficient consistency in a movement before it is progressed.

Second, you as coach need to keep both the progression principle and the appropriate variations in mind as you add complexity to the program. For

---

[68] Vladimir Zatsiorsky and William Kraemer, *Science and Practice of Strength Training*, 2nd revised edition, Champaign US, Human Kinetics, 2007.

example, going from a goblet squat to a single-arm rack squat requires the added skill of a clean as well as the demands imposed on the asymmetrical loading of the kettlebell.

As your clients acquire new skills, you are able to train more complex manoeuvres such as the rack squat. Unfortunately, trainers often fail to acknowledge a client's newly acquired skills, missing out on a great opportunity to boost positivity – and your own stature. As a trainer, you should highly value and feel great personal satisfaction when your client rises to the challenge of added complexity or acquires a new skill.

Celebrate these small but significant key wins and you will see levels of engagement from your client sky rocket!

Rest and recovery sessions

Clients are athletes who need your programming guidance and structure, but they also need to be educated on the importance of rest and recovery (R&R). Insufficient R&R leads to overtraining, which not only prevents them from achieving their fitness goals but is also detrimental to their health and wellbeing.

It is your responsibility to ensure your client receives proper R&R, which does not mean to simply have them do nothing for a brief period. Instead, make the R&R time more productive by empowering your group to listen to and feel how their body responds to each session. In other words, bring the mind-body connection into play.

Some R&R methods are:

- Yoga
- Remedial massage
- SMR (foam rolling techniques)
- Meditation and mindfulness
- Deep breathing techniques

As you can see from this discussion on workout types and programming principles, there's a lot to consider when it comes to programming the right kind of microcycle/individual session for your client. Coaching a client to fitness success is more than just giving them a hard session – it involves comprehensive strategies and techniques to bring together a balanced approach to fitness. But it is something that every committed coach can become skilled at with patience and practice.

Program review

Reviewing the success of a program is an essential part of the programming system. In the Adaptive FTS, we recommend reviewing your program at the end of each mesocycle.

We start with evaluation and we finish with evaluation – quantifiable results! This is an opportunity not only to assess your clients' progress, but also to involve them in the review and consultation process for planning out the next mesocycle.

- What are the fitness test results?
- Did the client stick to their plan?
- What exercises did they like/dislike or best respond to?
- Was the program too easy/too hard?
- Was training frequency achievable?
- What fitness tests are applicable to the next mesocycle?
- Take photos if appropriate
- Did they reach their milestone?

Remember that you are assessing whether the client achieved the training adaptation from that preceding mesocycle. The overall macrocycle (or even longer-term) goal could be to lose fat, but, more importantly, did your client 'Restore Function and Develop Proper Movement Patterns'?

Do your quantifiable results match this target? If yes, then celebrate! You and your client are on track and ready to begin the next mesocycle.

Reaching milestones will instil more trust and generate more enthusiasm to keep going; clients see that the system is working, and the vision of their end goal is looking real.

Above all, keep the end in mind, which is to move with purpose.

ONLINE RESOURCE: We have included a bunch of great additional programming resources'. Visit our resource link to find out more – http://functionaltraininginstitute.com/book-resources/

The Adaptive FTS Program

Now that we have established an understanding of periodisation, program types and key principles, it is time for us to design and build a program based on the Adaptive Functional Training System.

Note: As with any training plan, we need to customise the program for each individual based on a thorough assessment process as we have already explored in Part 2, *Assess with Purpose*. To that end, the program provided here is based on a hypothetical client and is designed to give you a head start in the formulation of your own training plan for your clients.

Background information

THE MESOCYCLES

This a twelve-week periodised training program. It has three mesocycles (phases) that are each four weeks long. During each phase, there are specific training qualities to focus on and they are in order according to standard principles of programming and periodisation, starting with the foundations of building muscle and cardiovascular endurance and then progressing through to strength, power and speed.

The training qualities or objectives for each mesocycle are as follows:

- **Phase 1** = Restore function, improve muscle endurance, improve cardiovascular endurance.
- **Phase 2** = Increase muscle size, develop better neural control, increase metabolic output and improve tolerance for more intense exercises to follow in the next cycle.
- **Phase 3** = Increase strength and power.

MICROCYCLES

In this case the microcycle, being one week long, is typical of most training programs. There are three training sessions for each microcycle. This is therefore a 3-day-per-week training plan. However, it is possible to make it into a 4-day-per-week training plan, and that is probably more suitable for many of us.

Here's how to convert it to a 4-day-per-week training cycle:

Within each training session there are different components such as warm-up, core, skill, movement/strength and conditioning. You could take the last component of each of the workouts (which is usually conditioning) and make this into another workout day on its own.

Here's an example of how you can manipulate the training plan from three days to four days per week:

3-day per week

	Monday	Tuesday	Wednesday	Thursday	Friday
Week 1	Day 1 Entire Session 1	Rest	Day 2 Entire Session 2	Rest	Day 3 Entire Session 3

4-day per week

	Monday	Tuesday	Wednesday	Thursday	Friday
Week 1	Day 1 Entire Session 1	Day 2 Session 2 without the conditioning	Rest	Day 3 Conditioning components from session 2 and 3	Day 4 Session 3 without the conditioning

EXERCISE SELECTION

Over 90% of the exercises selected within the program are what we teach in the FTI Master Functional Trainer (MFT) course.[69] These include exercises from the following workshops:

1. Mobility
2. Suspended Fitness Training (SFT)
3. Powerbags/Sandbags (SB)
4. Kettlebells (KB)
5. Battle ropes (BR)

As you'll recognise, these align with our 5 Pillars.

You will see that we don't include barbell training in this program. Barbells are most certainly a staple training tool that warrant selection in virtually any training program; however, we have opted to stick with the training tools from our 5 Pillars so that coaches learn to exploit the true versatility of these tools. If you execute this program correctly, there is no doubt that you will gain whole new levels of cardiovascular output and strength.

Sample Adaptive FTS 12-Week Program

Over the next few pages you will find a sample FTI 12-week program. To this point we have been theorising about programming and in particular how the adaptive FTS system may mould into an effective way of structuring programs. That is why we thought adding a comprehensive sample will serve to demonstrate how this structured programming looks and equally to inspire you to begin thinking precisely in this manner.

ONLINE RESOURCE: To get your free template visit our resource link – http://functionaltraininginstitute.com/book-resources/

---

69   You can find out more about this certification at: functionaltraininginstitute.com/course/master-functional-trainer/

DAY 1

Mobility Focus: Ankles, Hips

Skill Focus: Single-leg Hinge

Training focus
1. Restore Function
2. Develop Function
3. Build Muscle Endurance

Tissue quality – release
1. Gastrocnemius
2. Abductors
3. Quadriceps
4. ITB / Hip Flexors
5. Glutes

Movement prep
1. Standing Knee To Wall (Ankle)
2. Pulsed Hip Flexor Mobilisation
3. Rectus Femoris Mobilisation
4. Sumo Goblet Squat – Hip Abduction / Ext Rotation
5. Banded Squat / Banded Clams

MFT Phase 1

	Week 1 Date:				Week 2 Date:				Week 3 Date:				Week 4 Date:			
Core/skill	Target		Actual		Progression	Target	Actual		Progression	Target	Actual		Progression	Target	Actual	
	Sets	Reps	Sets	Reps		Sets	Reps	Sets	Reps		Sets	Reps	Sets	Reps	Sets	Reps
A1 Kneeling SB Hinge	3 x 30 sec				Staggered Stance Deadlift								Single-leg Deadlift			
A2 Front Plank	3 x 30 sec				SFS Plank								SFS Plank			
Movement Focus	Target		Actual			Target		Actual			Target		Actual		Target	Actual
	Sets	Reps	Sets	Reps		Sets	Reps	Sets	Reps		Sets	Reps	Sets	Reps	Sets	Reps
B1 SB Bear Hug Squat	2	15				3	15				3	12			3	12
B2 Suspended Row	2	15				3	15				3	10			3	10
C1 SB Deadlift / High Pull	2	15				3	15				3	12			3	12
C2 Suspended Push-up	2	15				3	15				3	10			3	10
Conditioning	Target		Actual			Target		Actual			Target		Actual		Target	Actual
AMRAP	2 rounds					3 rounds					3 rounds				> 3 rounds	
Suspended Biceps Curl x 8	7 mins					7 min					7 min				7 min	
Suspended Triceps Press x 8						x 10					x 12					
Run x 300m						x 10					x 12					

LET THE JOURNEY BEGIN

DAY 2

Mobility Focus: Shoulders
Skill Focus: SB + KB Clean and Press

MFT Phase 1

	Week 1				Week 2				Week 3				Week 4			
Date:					Date:				Date:				Date:			
Core/skill	Target		Actual		Progression		Actual		Progression		Actual		Progression		Actual	
A1 KB Two-Hand Clean	3 x 30 sec				KB Single-Arm Dead Clean				KB Swing Swing Clean				KB Clean			
2 A2 SB Overhead Walk	3 x 30 sec								KB Single Overhead Walk							
Movement Focus	Target		Actual		Target		Actual		Target		Actual		Target		Actual	
	Sets	Reps	Sets	Reps	Sets	Reps	Sets	Reps	Sets	Reps	Sets	Reps	Sets	Reps	Sets	Reps
B1 SB Front Squat	2	15			3	15			3	12			3	12		
B2 Assisted Pull-up / Lat Pull-Down	2	8			3	8			3	10			3	10		
C1 KB Swing	2	15			3	15			3	20			3	15ES		
C2 KB Two-Hand Press / Single Press	3	15			3	10ES			3	10ES			3	10ES		
Conditioning	Target		Actual		Target		Actual		Target		Actual		Target		Actual	
KB Complex	2 rounds				3 rounds				3 rounds				3 rounds			
KB Figure of 8 x 8ES					x 10				x 12							
KB Row x 8ES					x 10				x 12							
KB Halo x 8ES																
KB Lunge x 8 ES																

Training focus
1. Restore Function
2. Develop Function
3. Build Muscle Endurance

Tissue quality – release
1. Pecs
2. External Rotators
3. Lats
4. Triceps
5. Upper Traps

Movement prep
1. Kneeling Lat Dorsi Mobilisation
2. Forearm Wall Slide
3. Scapular Wall Slide
4. Sleeper Mobilisation
5. Scapular Push-up

TECHNIQUE IS PRIMARY

DAY 3

Mobility Focus:
Thoracic Extension / Rotation

Skill Focus: Turkish Get-up

Training focus
1. Restore Function
2. Develop Function
3. Build Muscle Endurance

Tissue quality – release
1. T-Spine / Rhomboids / Traps
2. Lats
3. Triceps
4. Pecs

Movement prep
1. Foam Roller T-Spine Breathing Extension
2. Bent-over Rotation
3. Quadruped Extention / Rotation
4. Kneeling bench breathing / Stretch
5. Down Dog to Updog (Pike Mobilisation)

MFT Phase 1

	Week 1				Week 2				Week 3				Week 4			
Date:					Date:				Date:				Date:			
	Target		Actual		Progression	Target		Actual		Progression	Target		Actual		Progression	Target		Actual	
Core/skill	Sets	Reps	Sets	Reps		Sets	Reps	Sets	Reps		Sets	Reps	Sets	Reps		Sets	Reps	Sets	Reps
A1 KB Low Windmill	3 x 30sec ES				KB High Windmill					KB TGU									
A2 SB Overhead Kneel to Stand	3 x 30sec ES																		
A3 BW 1/2 TGU	3 x 30sec ES				Add Leg Sweep					BW TGU									
Movement Focus	Sets	Reps	Sets	Reps		Sets	Reps	Sets	Reps		Sets	Reps	Sets	Reps		Sets	Reps	Sets	Reps
B1 SB Staggered Stance Squat	2	10ES				3	15				3	12				3	12		
B2 SB Bent-over Row	2	15				3	15				3	10				3	10		
C1 Double KB Step-ups	2	10ES				3	10ES				3	20				3	8ES		
C2 Double KB Floor Press	2	15				3	10				3	10ES				3	10		
Conditioning	Target		Actual			Target		Actual			Target		Actual			Target		Actual	
Circuit 30 sec: 15 sec x 3 rounds	2 rounds					3 rounds					3 rounds					> 3 rounds			
Suspended Hamstring Curl																			
Burpees																			
Shuttle Runs - 5 m distance																			

TRAINING INTENT IS ALL-IMPORTANT

DAY 1 — MFT Phase 2

Mobility Focus: Thoracic / Shoulders
Skill Focus: Double KB Jerk

Training focus
1. Functional Hypertrophy
2. Upper Body
3. Girevoy Conditioning

Core/skill

	Week 1 Date:			Week 2 Date:			Week 3 Date:			Week 4 Date:		
	Target	Actual		Progression	Actual		Progression	Actual		Progression	Actual	
		Sets	Reps		Sets	Reps		Sets	Reps		Sets	Reps
A1 KB Pistol Press	2 x 8ES						KB High Windmill			KB Uppercuts		
A2 Double KB Renegade Row	2 x 8ES											
KB 1/2 TGU	2 x 8ES						BW TGU			KB TGU 2 x 3ES		

Functional Hypertrophy

	Target		Actual		Target		Actual		Target		Actual		Target		Actual	
	Sets	Reps	Sets	Reps	Sets	Reps	Sets	Reps	Sets	Reps	Sets	Reps	Sets	Reps	Sets	Reps
B1 SB Weighted Push-ups	3	10			3	12			4	10			2	8		
B2 KB Single-leg Dead Lift	3	8ES			3	10ES			4	8ES			2	8ES		
C1 Double KB Alternating Press	3	10ES			3	12ES			4	8ES			2	8ES		
C2 KB Row	3	10ES			3	12ES			4	10ES			2	8ES		

Girevoy Conditioning

	Target	Actual	Target	Actual	Target	Actual	Target	Actual
	1 round		1 round		1 round		2 rounds	
Double KB Jerk	8 x 1 min, 1 min rest		10 x 1 min, 1 min rest		Pyramid kg*		Pyramid kg*	
					12 kg x 2 min		12 kg x 30 reps	
					16 kg x 90 sec		16 kg x 20 reps	
					20 kg x 1 min		20 kg x 10 reps	
					24 kg x 30 sec		24 kg x 5 reps	

* Weight in kg is based on 16 kg = 100%. Adjust for you

Tissue quality – release
1. T-Spine / Rhomboids / Traps
2. Lats
3. Triceps
4. Pecs

Mobility / Movement prep
1. Foam Roller T-Spine Breathing Extension
2. Bent-over Rotation
3. Quadruped Extention / Rotation
4. Kneeling bench breathing / Stretch
5. Down Dog to Updog (Pike Mobilisation)

Notes:
Aim to hit a load that matches the reps i.e. 10 reps would be about your 11–13RM

Pyramid W3 complete just once through

Pyramid W4 complete 40, 30, 20, 10, 10, 20, 30

Pyramid W3 + W4. Strict 2 min rest between sets

May need to do Girevoy on different day
Don't overdo

DAY 2

Mobility Focus: Shoulders / Thoracic
Skill Focus: KB Snatch

MFT Phase 2

		Date:				Date:				Date:				Date:			
		Week 1				Week 2				Week 3				Week 4			
		Target		Progression		Target		Progression		Target		Progression		Target		Progression	
Training focus	**Core/skill**	Work	Rest	Actual	Rounds	Work	Rest	Actual	Rounds	Work	Rest	Actual	Rounds	Work	Rest	Actual	Rounds
1 Grip Strength	A1 Double KB Farmers Walk	3 x 50 m				DKB Rack Carry				DKB Farmer Carry				DKB Rack Carry			
2 General Physical Preparation	A2 KB Squat High Swing	3 x 12															
3 Girevoy Conditioning	**GPP**																
	B1 SB Cleans	3 sec	15 sec		3	45 sec	15 sec		2	60 sec	0		2	30 sec	30 sec		3
Tissue quality – release	B2 SB Zercher Squats																
1 Pecs	B3 SB Push Press																
2 External Rotators	B4 Suspended Row																
3 Lats	B5 Suspended Push-ups																
4 Triceps	B6 Suspended Oblique Knee Tucks																
5 Upper Traps	B7 KB Side Swing																
Mobility / Movement prep	B8 KB Alternating High Pull																
1 Kneeling Lat Dorsi Mobilisation	B9 KB Halo																
2 Forearm Wall Slide	B10 Shuttle Runs – 5 m distance																
3 Scapular Wall Slide	**Girevoy Conditioning**	Target		Actual		Target		Actual		Target		Actual		Target		Actual	
4 Sleeper Mobilisation		20 Sets ES				16 Sets ES				24 Sets ES				12 Sets ES			
5 Scapular Push-up	**Target – Men 16kg / Women 10kg**	EMOM @ 30 sec				EMOM @ 30 sec				EMOM @ 30 sec				EMOM @ 30 sec			
Notes:	D1 Snatch – Left hand x 7	Dead Snatch x 6				Swing then Snatch x 3				Snatch x 6				Snatch x 7			
	D1 Snatch – Right hand x 7	Dead Snatch x 6				Swing then Snatch x 3				Snatch x 6				Snatch x 7			

Notes:

GPP goal is to reach anaerobic threshold i.e. 85% HR max and maintain this zone for as long as you can

Rest 3 min between GPP rounds

Girevoy: alternate hands every 30 sec

Girevoy can be done on a separate day as the entire session might be too much

DAY 3

MFT Phase 2

Mobility Focus: **Ankles, Hips**
Skill Focus: **Double KB Cleans**

Training focus
1. Functional Hypertrophy
2. Lower Body
3. Metabolic Conditioning

Tissue quality – release
1. Gastrocnemius
2. Abductors
3. Quadriceps
4. ITB / hip flexors
5. Glutes

Mobility / Movement preparation
1. Standing Knee To Wall (Ankle)
2. Pulsed Hip Flexor Mobilisation
3. Rectus Femoris Mobilisation
4. Sumo Goblet Squat – Hip Abduction / Ext Rotation
5. Banded Squat / Banded Clams

Notes:
Aim to hit a load that matches the reps
i.e. 10 reps would be about your 11–13RM
RFE = Rear Foot Elevated (or Bulgarian)

	Week 1 Date:				Week 2 Date:				Week 3 Date:				Week 4 Date:			
	Target		Actual		Target	Progression	Actual		Target	Progression	Actual		Target	Progression	Actual	
Core/skill	Sets	Reps	Sets	Reps	Sets	Reps	Sets	Reps	Sets	Reps	Sets	Reps	Sets	Reps	Sets	Reps
A1 Dowel Overhead Squat	2 x 8															
A2 Hand Walkout	2 x 8															
A3 BW Split Squat	2 x 8ES															
A4 KB Dead Clean	2 x 8ES															
Functional Hypertrophy																
B1 Double KB Cleans	3	12			3	10			4	8			2	10		
B2 Double KB Front Squat	3	8ES			3	10ES			4	10ES			2	10ES		
C1 Double KB RFE Split Squat	3	12ES			3	10ES			4	8ES			2	8ES		
C2 SB Zercher Good Mornings	3	15			3	15			3	12			2	12		
Metabolic Conditioning	Target		Actual		Target		Actual		Target		Actual		Target		Actual	
Tabata 20:10 D1 to D4 twice through = 1 Round	2 rounds				3 rounds				3 rounds				2 rounds			
D1 Double KB Alternating High Pulls																
D2 Battling Rope Slams																
D3 Suspended Ice Skater																
D4 Battling Rope Bull Whips																

DAY 1

Mobility Focus: Ankles, Hips
Skill Focus: Double KB Squat

MFT Phase 3

	Week 1				Week 2				Week 3				Week 4			
Date:																
	Progression				Progression				Progression				Progression			
	Target		Actual		Target		Actual		Target		Actual		Target		Actual	
Movement prep	Sets	Reps	Sets	Reps	Sets	Reps	Sets	Reps	Sets	Reps	Sets	Reps	Sets	Reps	Sets	Reps
A1 Frog Squat	3 x 30 sec															
A2 Bear Crawl	3 x 30 sec															
A3 Inch Worm	3 x 30 sec															
Power	Target		Actual		Target		Actual		Target		Actual		Target		Actual	
	Sets	Reps	Sets	Reps	Sets	Reps	Sets	Reps	Sets	Reps	Sets	Reps	Sets	Reps	Sets	Reps
B1 Box Jumps	3	8			4	6			5	5			3	4		
Strength	Target		Actual		Target		Actual		Target		Actual		Target		Actual	
	Sets	Reps	Sets	Reps	Sets	Reps	Sets	Reps	Sets	Reps	Sets	Reps	Sets	Reps	Sets	Reps
C1 Double KB Squat	3	5			4	4ES			5	3ES			4	5,3,1,1		
C1 Weighted Chin-up	3	8			4	6			5	4			4	2		
Trunk	Target		Actual		Target		Actual		Target		Actual		Target		Actual	
	Sets	Reps	Sets	Reps	Sets	Reps	Sets	Reps	Sets	Reps	Sets	Reps	Sets	Reps	Sets	Reps
D1 Double KB Windmill	3	10ES			3	10ES			4	10ES			2	8ES		
Conditioning	Target		Actual		Target		Actual		Target		Actual		Target		Actual	
	5 rounds				3 rounds				3 rounds				2 rounds			

Battling Rope. 10 sec work :50 sec rest. Explosive

E1 Bull Whip
E2 Alternating Waves
E3 Double Wave Slams
E4 Waves with Jumping Split Squats

Training focus

1. Vertical Jump
2. Lower Body Strength

Tissue quality – release

1. Gastrocnemius
2. Abductors
3. Quadriceps
4. ITB / hip flexors
5. Glutes

Mobility / Movement prep

1. Standing Knee To Wall (Ankle)
2. Pulsed Hip Flexor Mobilisation
3. Rectus Femoris Mobilisation
4. Sumo Goblet Squat – Hip Abduction / Ext Rotation
5. Banded Squat / Banded Clams

Notes:

Rest as needed between sets.
Power and Strength. Require at least 2 min rest between sets.
Always lift fast in concentric phase
Hold 2 seconds in bottom position of squat
Perform BR waves explosively to warrant rest ratio

DAY 2

Mobility Focus: Shoulders / Thoracic

Skill Focus: KB Alternating Press

MFT Phase 3

		Week 1				Week 2				Week 3				Week 4			
		Date:				Date:				Date:				Date:			
		Target		Actual		Progression		Actual		Progression		Actual		Progression		Actual	
Movement prep				Sets	Reps	Sets	Reps	Sets	Reps	Sets	Reps	Sets	Reps	Sets	Reps	Sets	Reps
	A1 Frog Squat	3 x 10															
	A2 Bear Crawl	3 x 10															
	A3 KB Row	3 x 10ES															
Power		Target		Actual		Target		Actual		Target		Actual		Target		Actual	
		Sets	Reps	Sets	Reps	Sets	Reps	Sets	Reps	Sets	Reps	Sets	Reps	Sets	Reps	Sets	Reps
	B1 Plyometric Push-ups	3	6			3	6			4	6			2	5		
	B2 Suspended Stability Lunge Jump	3	10			3	10			4	10			2	10		
Strength		Target		Actual		Target		Actual		Target		Actual		Target		Actual	
		Sets	Reps	Sets	Reps	Sets	Reps	Sets	Reps	Sets	Reps	Sets	Reps	Sets	Reps	Sets	Reps
	C1 Double KB Alternating Press	4	6ES			5	5ES			6	4ES			4	3ES		
	C2 Double KB Single-leg Deadlift	4	6ES			5	6ES			6	8ES			4	6ES		
Trunk		Target		Actual		Target		Actual		Target		Actual		Target		Actual	
		Sets	Reps	Sets	Reps	Sets	Reps	Sets	Reps	Sets	Reps	Sets	Reps	Sets	Reps	Sets	Reps
	D1 Double KB Windmill	3	10ES			3	10ES			4	10ES			2	8ES		
Conditioning		Target		Actual		Target		Actual		Target		Actual		Target		Actual	
	Battling Rope Endurance					3 rounds				3 rounds				2 rounds			
	E1 Battling Rope waves	8 sets of 1 min 2 min rest				6 sets of 90 sec 2 min rest				5 sets of 2 min 2 min rest				3 sets of 3 min 3 min rest			

Training focus
1. Push Power
2. Upper Push Strength
3. Battling Rope Endurance

Tissue quality – release
1. Pecs
2. External Rotators
3. Lats
4. Triceps
5. Upper Traps

Mobility / Movement prep
1. Kneeling Lat Dorsi Mobilisation
2. Forearm Wall Slide
3. Scapular Wall Slide
4. Sleeper Mobilisation
5. Scapular Push-up

Notes:
Rest as needed between sets.
Power and Strength. Require at least 2 min rest between sets.
Always lift fast in concentric phase
Battling Rope aim is to keep constant velocity to the anchorpoint for entire time allocated to each set

DAY 3

Mobility Focus: Thoracic / Shoulders

Skill Focus: TGU

Training focus
1. Proprioception
2. Strength
3. Sprint

Tissue quality – release
1. T-Spine / Rhomboids / Traps
2. Lats
3. Triceps
4. Pecs

Mobility / Movement prep
1. Foam Roller T-Spine Breathing Extension
2. Kneeling Lat Dorsi Mobilisation
3. Quadruped Extention / Rotation
4. Kneeling bench breathing/Stretch
5. Down Dog to Updog (Pike Mobilisation)

MFT Phase 3

	Week 1 Date:				Week 2 Date:				Week 3 Date:				Week 4 Date:			
Movement prep	Target		Actual		Progression		Actual		Progression		Actual		Progression		Actual	
	Sets	Reps	Sets	Reps	Sets	Reps	Sets	Reps	Sets	Reps	Sets	Reps	Sets	Reps	Sets	Reps
A1 Duck Walk	3 x 30 sec															
A2 Get Down Get Up	3 x 30 sec															
A3 KB Snatch	3 x 30 sec ES															
Power	Target		Actual		Target		Actual		Target		Actual		Target		Actual	
	Sets	Reps	Sets	Reps	Sets	Reps	Sets	Reps	Sets	Reps	Sets	Reps	Sets	Reps	Sets	Reps
B1 Double KB Jerk	3	5			3	4			4	3			2	3		
B2 KB Snatch	3	6ES			3	6ES			4	5ES			2	6ES		
Strength	Target		Actual		Target		Actual		Target		Actual		Target		Actual	
	Sets	Reps	Sets	Reps	Sets	Reps	Sets	Reps	Sets	Reps	Sets	Reps	Sets	Reps	Sets	Reps
C1 TGU	4	5ES			5	4ES			5	3ES			4	5,3,1,1		
C1 Weighted Push-up with SB	4	8			5	6			5	4			4	10ES		
Trunk	Target		Actual		Target		Actual		Target		Actual		Target		Actual	
	Sets	Reps	Sets	Reps	Sets	Reps	Sets	Reps	Sets	Reps	Sets	Reps	Sets	Reps	Sets	Reps
D1 Suspended Side Plank	3	30 sec ES			3	30 sec ES			4	40 sec ES			2	40 sec ES		
D2 Double KB Front Squat	3	8ES			3	10ES			4	8ES			2	10ES		
Conditioning	Target		Actual		Target		Actual		Target		Actual		Target		Actual	
Battling Rope Endurance					3 rounds				3 rounds				2 rounds			
Sprint	8 x 60 m				2 min rest				8 x 50 m – hill				8 x 20 m			
Sled Push																

Notes:
Rest as needed between sets.
Power and Strength. Require at least 2 min rest between sets.
Always lift fast in concentric phase
Sprint can be completed by other locomotion options if not suitable e.g. rowing, bike, air dyne
Rest minimum 3 min between sprints

Adapting the program for different clients

It's impossible to develop one program that will be suitable for all coaches and their clients. Here are some circumstances that you may need to work around, and some advice for how to improvise and be flexible:

- **Not having access to all of the available tools.** For example, when doing strength work with heavy kettlebell front squats, maybe you are limited by how heavy your kettlebells are. In this situation, you could resort to using a barbell.

- **The program progresses too fast for a client.** There are many reasons why this could be; perhaps a client has a lesser training history or perhaps they have mobility issues that prevent fast progression of exercises. The simple answer is to stick with the same phase of training until complete competency has been gained before moving onto the next. That may mean going through the same phase two to three times.

- **Sessions are too long or there is too much work in each session for your client's level of fitness.** Refer back to microcycles above and how to turn this program into a 4-day-per-week program.

- **There's an injury to work around.** An example could be a shoulder impingement that prevents any overhead movement. You will be required to again improvise by changing this exercise. The two options available are to switch to more appropriate strength exercise (for example, from a kettlebell overhead press to a kettlebell floor press), or you could swap the exercise for rehab work to address the problem of that impingement (for example, external rotator and stabiliser activations).

- **You're unsure about a deload week.** These weeks are important to refresh the mind and body. Typical programs have deload weeks every four weeks, and we have included that in this program as well. But the reality is that it's only necessary if the preceding weeks have been very intense and the stress on the individual is rather high. It may well be that an individual is feeling awesome in week four and is ready to hit their peak, so there is no need to hold them back. Many individuals may have external stressors such as work and family pressures and mental health issues, and all of these stressors play a part in the overall training load that someone can handle. It will be up to you as a coach to determine stress loads through feedback from your client, both verbally and physically, as you note their performance in each session. Most regular clients do not train frequently or intensely enough to warrant a full deload where a trained professional athlete would. It's a complex subject, but something to consider.

Next steps

Our aim with this book has been to show you a functional training system that is progressive, fluid and adaptive – one you can implement in your own purpose driven coaching practice. From exploring the importance of coaching and assessing techniques to the need for smart programming, the Adaptive Functional Training System provides a framework for trainers and coaches to build a foundation of purpose driven movement with the capacity to keep evolving and challenging our understanding of exercise prescription.

Functional training is not an elite methodology, but a form of training suitable for everyone. As we've argued, we believe functional training methods must not exclude certain people from the fun, dynamism and challenge that is inherent to this form of movement. In the Adaptive FTS, the tools we choose are specific to the client's needs because the outcome for the client is what matters. Instead of being random in the way we select and program in any particular functional exercise, we have created a logical, flexible and progressive system for all trainers and coaches – a system that has benefited thousands of trainers globally so far and will continue to impact thousands more to come.

We have shown you what it takes to understand truly functional training – purpose driven movement – and incorporate it into your training practice. We've unpacked how you can form your own unique coaching style and refine your coaching technique, become a champion for injury awareness and prevention, integrate functional tools and exercises into your training in a gradual and deliberate way and bring it all together in programs that really deliver for your clients – and yourself.

Now it's over to you to implement what you've learned.

The fact that you have worked your way through this book demonstrates your personal commitment to the kind of functional training that will make a difference in the lives of your clients.

The question you need to ask yourself now is, 'What is the next step in your journey toward being a purpose driven coach?'

Perhaps you want to:

- Put more thought into what you stand for as a coach and how to bring this into your day-to-day training?
- Get more confident in your ability to assess movement patterns for injury, educate your clients and improve their injury outcomes?
- Build your own technical training skills from the ground up, or learn how to coach the exercises/use the tools showcased in our pillars with more confidence?
- Take your programming skills to the next level?

We have many recommended books, FTI courses and partnering resources to help you develop in each of these areas. We suggest you start by checking out our *Resource Pool* on page the next page as you consider your next steps.

The best coaches recognise that true mastery is not a static thing but involves continual learning and growth. At FTI, we strive to understand human movement more deeply so that we can truly train, coach and live with purpose. We invite you to join us.

Resource pool

Coach with Purpose

RECOMMENDED READING

Covey, Stephen. *The Seven Habits of Highly Effective People*. New York, Fireside Books, 2004.

Csikszentmihalyi, Mihaly. *Flow*. New York, Harper, 2008.

Dweck, Carol. *Mindset: The New Psychology of Success*. New York, Random House, 2016.

Gallwey, W Timothy. *The Inner Game of Tennis*. London, Pan Macmillan, 2015.

Godan, Seth. *Tribes: We Need You to Lead Us*. New York, Penguin, 2008.

Langer, Ellen. *Mindfulness*. Cambridge MA, Westview, 1990.

Pink, Daniel H. *Drive: The Surprising Truth about What Motivates Us*. Edinburgh, Canongate, 2018.

Plummer, Thomas. *The Soul of a Trainer: You Were Born to Change the World*. On Target Publications, 2018.

Sinek, Simon. *Start with Why: How Great Leaders Inspire Everyone to Take Action*. London, Penguin, 2018.

Sugarman, Roy. *Client Centered Training: A Trainer and Coach's Guide to Motivating Clients*. PTA Global, 2014.

Wulf, Gabriele. *Attention and Motor Skill Learning*. Champaign IL, Human Kinetics, 2007.

USEFUL WEB LINKS

Self Determination Theory www.sdt.org

Thomas Plummer www.thomasplummer.blog

Training for Warriors www.trainingforwarriors.com

Assess with Purpose

RECOMMENDED READING

Anderson, Tim and Geoff Neupert. *Original Strength*. US, Xulon Press, 2014.

Cook, Gray. *Movement: Functional Movement Systems*. Aptos CA, On Target Publications, 2010.

McGill, Stuart. *Low Back Disorders*, Champaign IL, Human Kinetics, 2015.

USEFUL WEB LINKS

Rehab Trainer www.Rehabtrainer.com.au

Functional Movement Screens www.functionalmovement.com

Move with Purpose

RECOMMENDED READING

Bompa, Tudor and Carlo Buzzicheli. *Periodization Training for Sports*. 3rd edition. Champaign IL, Human Kinetics, 2015.

Calais-Germain, Blandine. *Anatomy of Movement*. Revised edition. Pennington US, Princeton Book Company, 2008.

Chek, Paul. *How to Eat, Move and Be Healthy*. Vista, CHEK Institute, 2004.

Chu, Donald A. *Jumping into Plyometrics*. Champaign IL, Human Kinetics, 1998.

Earls, James. *Born to Walk*. California, North Atlantic Books, 2014.

Jason Brumitt. *Core Assessment and Training*. Champaign IL, Human Kinetics, 2010.

Lee, Diane. *The Pelvic Girdle E-Book*. London, Elsevier, 2011.

Schleip, Robert et al., eds. *Fascia: The Tensional Network of the Human Body-E-Book*. London, Elsevier, 2012.

Schleip, Robert. *Fascial Fitness*. Chichester, Lotus, 2017.

USEFUL WEB LINKS

Animal Flow® www.animalflow.com

Dr Emily Splichel www.evidencebasedfitnessacademy.com

Original Strength www.originalstrength.net

John Brookfield www.powerropes.com

Joey Alvarado www.kjrevolution.com/about-joey-alvarado

Program with Purpose

RECOMMENDED READING

Bompa, Tudor and Gregory Haff, *Periodization: Theory and Methodology of Training*. Champaign IL, Human Kinetics, 2009.

Rooney, Martin. *Warrior Cardio: The Revolutionary Metabolic Training System for Burning Fat, Building Muscle and Getting Fit*. New York, HarperCollins, 2012.

Stone, Michael, Margaret Stone and William Sands. *Principles and Practice of Resistance Training*. Champaign US, Human Kinetics, 2007.

Zatsiorsky, Vladimir, and William Kraemer. *Science and Practice of Strength Training*. 2nd revised edition. Champaign US, Human Kinetics, 2007.

USEFUL WEB LINKS

PTA Global, 'Gears and intensity scale/model': www.ptacademy.edu.au/what-gear-do-you-drive-your-clients-in/

Alethiex www.alethiex.com

FTI Library www.alethiex.com/fti-library

FTI www.functionaltraininginstitute.com/learning-resources

FTI – Special offers for book readers

To access your free resources go to
http://functionaltraininginstitute.com/book-resources/

Redeem 20% off any course undertaken with FTI
with the following code: **FTIBook**

Visit **www.functionaltraininginstitute.com**

Find us on social media @FTIGlobal

www.ingramcontent.com/pod-product-compliance
Lightning Source LLC
Chambersburg PA
CBHW080245030426
42334CB00023BA/2702